# The Art of Traditional Thai Massage

by

**Asokananda**
(Harald Brust)

Editions Duang Kamol

© Copyright: Harald Brust, 1990. All rights reserved
© Copyright Photographs: Egbert Trogemann
3rd Edition, 1993

Editions Duang Kamol
G.P.O. Box 427
Bangkok 10501 Thailand
Tel. (662) 247-1001, 427-1031
Fax (662) 247-1033
Publisher Mr. Suk Soongswang
  Publisher's No. 6/1993 — 3,000

Typeset by COMSET Limited Partnership

Printed in Thailand by
  D. K. Printing House, Ltd.
  205/54-57 Ngamwongwan Rd.
  Bangkok 10210

Distributed by
  D.K. Today Co., Ltd.
  90/21-25 Rajprarop Road, Makkasan
  Bangkok 10400, Thailand
  Tel. (662) 245-5586, 247-1030
  Fax (662) 247-1033

All rights reserved. No part of this publication may be reproduced, stored in a retrieval system or transmitted in any form or by any means, electronic, mechanical, photocopying, recording or otherwise, without permission of the copyright owners.

The author and the publisher accept no responsibility for any loss, injury or damage sustained by anyone using this book.

ISBN 974-210-508-1

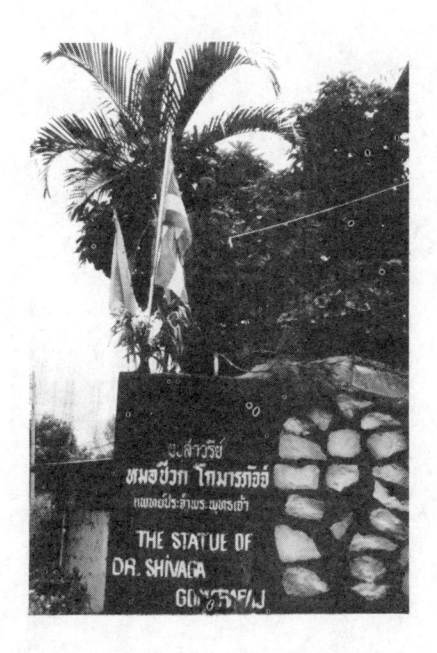

Statue in rememberance of the 'Founder' of Thai massage, the Indian Doctor Jivaka Kumar Bhaccha.

Entrance to the Massage Hospital of the "Foundation of Shivago Komarpaj", Chiang Mai, Thailand.

To my Teachers,

Chaiyuth Priyasith and Piched Boonthumme

To my Teachers,

Chaiyuth Priyasith and Piched Boonthumme

## Preface to the 3rd, revised edition

When this book was published at the end of the year 1990 it was the first book on traditional Thai massage in any Western language. Neither the publisher nor myself expected it to sell fast, as interest in this ancient form of healing massage seemed to be limited.

That a third edition of the book is necessary so soon proves us wrong, which is an encouraging sign that more and more people all over the world start to appreciate the art of 'Nuad Phaen Boran'. I use the opportunity of this new edition to revise the book, based on my own experiences of working with it and on suggestions by readers, although only minor changes were necessary. Thanks to all who took the trouble to write to me.

The book is now available in English, German and French, published by Duang Kamol, Bangkok. An Italian edition by Editione Mediterranee, Rome, is in preparation.

A big "Thank You" goes to my publisher, Khun Suk Soongswang, for fruitful and joyful cooperation.

Asokananda<br>
Chiang Mai, October 1992.

Thanks to all those involved in the realisation of this book:

Vera Lier, Lukas Ernst, Gabi Herr, Hazel Palmer, Nikki Veneti, Kusal Gupta, Prabhat Menon, "Major" Sintorn, Anagarika Munindra, Kumar Gupta, Bharat Mansata, Norbert Fiedler, Ulli Zeller, Peter Lanzendorf, Philippe Menu, and Shamir Roy.

The drawings, figures and diagrams are the work of Amal Bera, who is working for "Silence", a self-help organisation of deaf and dumb people in Calcutta. Anybody interested in more information on "Silence" may write to:

Silence, 2/1 A Monohar Pukur, Calcutta 700029, West Bengal, India; Tel. 42-7269

Cover : Pradip Acharya

Cartoons: Dr. Anja Lund

Photographs by: Egbert Trogemann, Düsseldorf, Tel.: (0211)38122

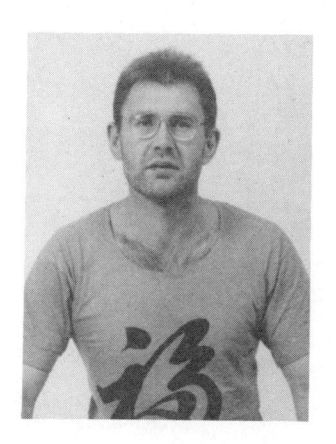

About the author:

Asokananda (Harald Brust, born in 1955 in West Germany) studied community development. Since 1978 he has made regular journeys to Asia, spending much time in India, Sri Lanka and Thailand teaching yoga, meditation and traditional massage. He was temporarily ordained as a Buddhist monk in Sri Lanka. He studied Thai massage at the Massage Hospital of the 'Foundation of Shivago Komarpaj' in Chiang Mai, Thailand.

# CONTENTS

## Part I
## Introduction

    1.1    The historical roots of Thai massage ............................................ 4

    1.2    The theoretical foundations of Thai massage ............................. 6

    1.3    The spirit of Thai massage ............................................................ 8

    1.4    Practical Thai massage ................................................................... 9

    1.5    Techniques and styles ................................................................... 11

    1.6    State of health of the patient ....................................................... 13

    1.7    How to learn? ................................................................................ 16

    1.8    The rules of a good Thai masseur ............................................. 17

## Part II
## A Whole-body Massage

    2.1    The front part of the body ......................................................... 21
           2.1.1   Feet ................................................................................ 23
           2.1.2   Energy lines on the legs ............................................. 31
           2.1.3   Exercises with one leg ................................................ 35
           2.1.4   Exercises with two legs .............................................. 48
           2.1.5   Stomach massage ........................................................ 54
           2.1.6   Chest and arms ............................................................ 58
           2.1.7   Hands and fingers ....................................................... 60

    2.2    The side position ......................................................................... 64
           2.2.1   Energy lines on the legs ............................................. 64
           2.2.2   Stretching ..................................................................... 65

    2.3    The back part of the body .......................................................... 69
           2.3.1   Feet and legs ................................................................ 69
           2.3.2   Lower back, spine, shoulders, and energy lines ............ 72
           2.3.3   "Cobra" stretches ........................................................ 75

- 2.4 The sitting position ..................................................... 77
  - 2.4.1 Sit-ups ................................................................ 77
  - 2.4.2 Arms, shoulders, and shoulder blades ........ 79
  - 2.4.3 Head and neck ................................................. 83
  - 2.4.4 Stretches .......................................................... 87

- 2.5 The face ........................................................................ 90

# Part III
# Appendices

- 3.1 The Theory of the 10 *Sen*:
  The energy mainlines of the Body .......................... 97

- 3.2 Therapy ...................................................................... 108
  - 3.2.1 Headache ....................................................... 109
  - 3.2.2 Knee pain ....................................................... 110
  - 3.2.3 Lower back pain ........................................... 111
  - 3.2.4 The use of oils and creams in therapy ....... 112
  - 3.2.5 Herbal treatment .......................................... 113

- 3.3 Places to learn traditional Thai massage ............ 114

- 3.4 Glossary of Thai, Pali and Sanskrit words .......... 117

- 3.5 Bibliography ............................................................. 118

- 3.6 Thai Bibliography ................................................... 119

# PART I

# INTRODUCTION

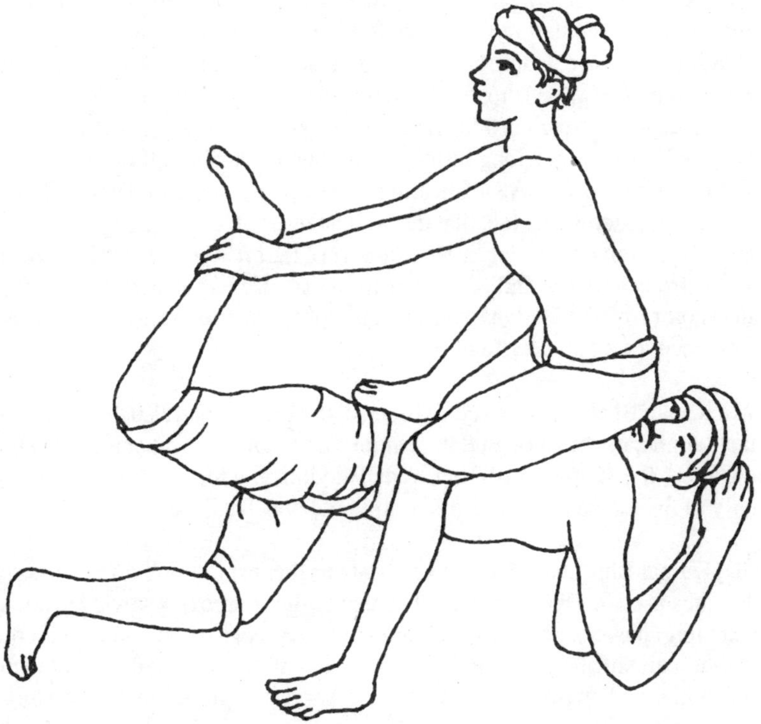

*Introduction*

*Illustration 1*
*Traditional Yoga massage*

"When any person is sick at Siam[1] he begins with causing his whole body to be moulded by one who is skilful herein, who gets upon the body of the sick person and tramples him under his feet."

    Simon de la Loubére, French liaison to the Thai Royal Court in Ayutthia, 1690.

---

[1] Thailand was called 'Siam' until the name was changed in 1949.

## 1.1 THE HISTORICAL ROOTS OF THAI MASSAGE

"Thai massage"—hearing those words, most people would automatically think of Bangkok's infamous nightlife and the massage parlours which offer services quite different from genuine massage. Thai massage unfortunately suffers from this reputation since very few foreign visitors arrive in Thailand already knowing that 'Traditional massage' is something totally different from the sort of thinly disguised prostitution found in Bangkok's parlours. Traditional Thai massage, or "Ancient Massage" (*nuad phaen boran*, as it is called in Thai), can look back at a long history of therapeutic healing. If one traces the evolution of the techniques of healing-massage practiced in Thailand, one discovers the astonishing fact that the earliest roots of Thai massage lie not in Thailand but in India. The legendary founder of the art is believed to have been a doctor from northern India. Known as Jivaka Kumar Bhaccha, he was a contemporary of the Buddha and personal physician to the Magadha King Bimbisara over 2,500 years ago.

Jivaka Kumar Bhaccha[1] was a close friend of the Buddha and also the physician of the Sangha, the order of Buddhist monks and nuns. He is mentioned in the Pali Canon, the scriptures of Theravada Buddhism, which is practiced today mainly in Sri Lanka, Burma, Laos, Cambodia and Thailand.

Jivaka Kumar Bhaccha is regarded not only as the inspiration for the massage techniques used in Thailand today, but also as the source of knowledge about the healing powers of herbs and minerals. Aspects of Indian Ayurvedic medicine can still be found in Thailand and—along with herbal treatment, steam baths and massage—comprise the services offered at the Massage Hospital run by the Foundation of Shivago Komarpaj in Chiang Mai in northern Thailand. And even today Kumar Bhaccha is respected and honoured by many Thais as the 'Father of Medicine'. Religious ceremonies (called Pujas in Pali and *bucha* in Thai) are conducted to remember him. A prayer in Pali language is chanted on these occasions: "Om namo Jivaka"—Jivaka, symbol of Cosmic Unity. "I venerate the compassionate Jivaka with good conduct..." These ceremonies, called *wai khru* in Thai, are still a daily ritual at the Massage Hospital in Chiang Mai and are performed twice a day.

Despite what is known about Kumar Bhaccha, much of the origins of Thai massage and traditional Thai medicine still remain obscure. It is believed that the teachings of Kumar Bhaccha reached what is now Thailand at the same time

---

[1] In Thailand you may come across some quite strange spellings of this name, such as Shivago Komarpaj, Shevaka Komarapatr, Shivago Kumar Baj. I have chosen to use the romanised version of the original Pali name.

*Introduction*

as Buddhism—as early as the 3rd or 2nd century B.C. It is unknown whether there was any indigenous form of massage in the region before that time. Equally unknown is to what extent Chinese concepts of acupuncture and acupressure (as well as other aspects of traditional medicine) had any theoretical and practical influence on the practice of massage in Thailand. Nowadays it is impossible to definitively answer such questions, since for centuries medical knowledge was transmitted almost entirely orally from teacher to student, following a teaching tradition also common in India. There is mention of massage in 17th century medical scriptures written on palm leaves in Pali language using Khmer (*khom*) script. These old texts seem to have been very important and were accorded respect similar to that bestowed on Buddhist scriptures. With the destruction of the old royal capital, Ayutthia, by Burmese invaders in 1767, most old texts were destroyed and are, sadly, gone forever. Only fragments survived and these were utilized in 1832 by King Rama III as the basis for the famous epigraphs at Phra Chetuphon Temple (popularly called Wat Pho) in Bangkok. The fragments were collected and compared and then carved in stone and placed into the walls of the temple. The diagrams (the cover of this book illustrates the sort of drawings that were used) and the corresponding explanations have their shortcomings. A publication of the 'Association of the Traditional Medical School in Thailand' published in 1977 in Thai language, presents " The Medical Texts which his Majesty King Rama III had engraved at Phra Chetuphon Temple (Wat Pho) in 2375 B.E. (1832 A.D.)." There are some contradictions between the diagrams and the explanatory notes; the diagrams lack ribs and vertebrae, and there are other inadequacies. But these graven texts are still a rich source—and the only source—for anyone interested in exploring the theoretical background of Thai massage. Altogether there are 60 figures, 30 depicting the front of the body and 30 the back. On the figures therapy-points are shown along the various energy lines called *Sen* in Thai; these lines form the primary theoretical basis of Thai massage. (These energy lines will be dealt with in more detail later on.) If one looks at these diagrams with a Western concept of anatomy in mind, they appear to be quite strange at best, the reason being that anatomy did not play a role in ancient Thai massage. Surgery was unknown in Thailand until quite recently, and dissection of corpses seems to have been banned in earlier Thai societies. Anatomical knowledge was therefore practically non-existent, and the massage-diagrams do not pretend to be physiologically accurate. They are only a schematic device to show the pattern of invisible energy lines and acupressure points—and their influence on the body and its functioning.

## 1.2 THE THEORETICAL FOUNDATION OF THAI MASSAGE

The theoretical foundation of Thai massage is based on the concept of invisible energy lines running through the body. Ten of these lines are especially important in Thai massage: 'The 10 *Sen*' or *sib sen*. The Indian origin and influence becomes obvious here since the background of this theory clearly lies in Yoga philosophy. Yoga philosophy states that life energy (called Prana) is absorbed with the air we breathe and with the food we eat. Along a network of energy lines, the Prana Nadis, the human being is then supplied with this vital energy. These energy lines are invisible and cannot be verified anatomically. They form a sort of 'second skin', a second body in addition to the physical body. Called Pranamaya Kosha or 'energy body', this second body is comprised of a multitude of energy lines, said to be 72,000. However that may be, there are many lines and out of this multitude Thai massage has selected 10 mainlines on which there are especially important acupressure points. Massaging these points makes it possible to treat certain diseases or to relieve pain.

The 10 *Sen* are sufficient to conduct practical treatment for the whole body and its internal organs. Western scientists are still puzzled by the fact that these lines and points do seem to have validity. Their existence can be validated practically by the curing of various diseases or, at the very least, by providing relief. These points can be thought of as 'windows' into the body. These 'windows' enable an exchange of cosmic energy through which the human body is maintained in an energy balance with the energy of the universe. Disturbances in the flow of energy result in an insufficient supply of Prana which will in turn lead to sickness. Working on the energy lines with massage can break the blockades, stimulate the free flow of Prana, and help to restore general well-being.

More or less the same theory is found in the Chinese systems of acupuncture and acupressure and also in the Japanese system of Shiatsu, which has evolved from Chinese models. (The energy lines in these systems are called meridians.) The origin of these systems is clouded in mystery. Some practitioners hold the opinion that their roots also lie in Indian Yoga philosophy, brought to China by Bodhidharma, the Indian saint who established Zen Buddhism in China—but such an origin is very much disputed by the Chinese. But whatever the origin of the Chinese teachings, there is little doubt but that the theory of the 10 *Sen* in Thai massage is based on the Indian transmission and not on the Chinese traditions. This relationship is manifested even in the terminology the Thais use, with many words quite obviously derived from Sanskrit, the ancient spiritual language of India. For example, the first three of the *Sen*—*Sen Sumana, Sen Ittha* and *Sen Pingkhala*—are not only linguistically cognate

*Introduction*

with Sushumna Nadi, Ida Nadi and Pingala Nadi, but these three Thai *Sen* follow paths very similar to the corresponding Prana Nadis. (A detailed description of the 10 *Sen* will be given in Section 3.1 of this book.)

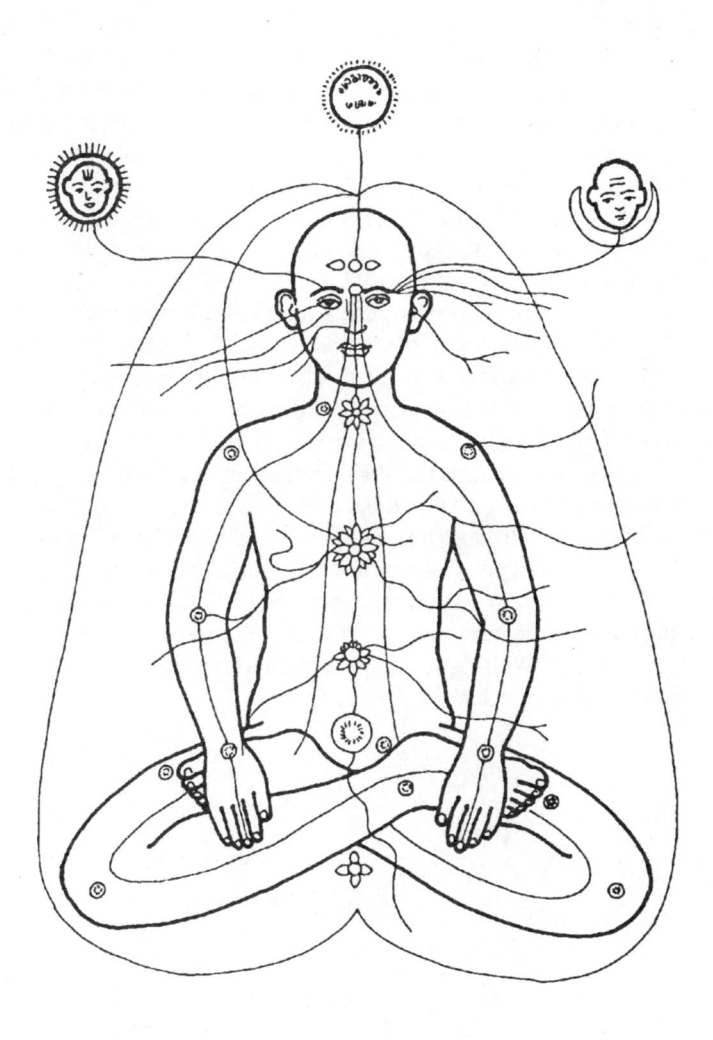

*Illustration 2*
*Simplified version of an ancient Yoga drawing. The drawing shows the running of some important energy lines (Prana Nadis) and the location of the main energy centers (Chakras) and some minor Chakras.*

## 1.3 THE SPIRIT OF THAI MASSAGE

Looking back at the tradition of Thai massage it is very clear that it was never seen as a mere job. Massage was always considered to be a spiritual practice closely connected with the teachings of the Buddha. Until fairly recently it was the *wat*, the temple, where massage was taught and practiced. Even today one of the most important massage schools in Thailand is at Wat Pho in Bangkok. The establishment of legitimate massage facilities outside of the temples is a recent development. The giving of massage was understood to be a physical application of Metta, the Pali (and Thai) word used in Theravada Buddhism to denote 'loving kindness'—and devoted masseurs still work in such a spirit today. A truly good masseur performs his art in a meditative mood. He starts with a Puja, a meditative prayer, to fully centre himself on the work, on the healing he is about to perform. And he works with full awareness, mindfulness and concentration. This is a difficult mental state to achieve and even in Thailand there are only a few masters skilled in that art. Most of these masters—and I was blessed with having two of them as my teachers—are deeply religious people who practice Buddhist meditation as well. For beginners it is important to keep this ideal in mind and to learn in that spirit. There is a world of a difference between a massage performed in a meditative mood and a massage done just as a job. Only the masseur working in a meditative mood will develop an intuition for the energy flow in the body and for the Prana lines. Only a spiritually aware masseur is able to treat different people according to their different needs. Without such higher consciousness, massage becomes mechanical and loses much of its power.

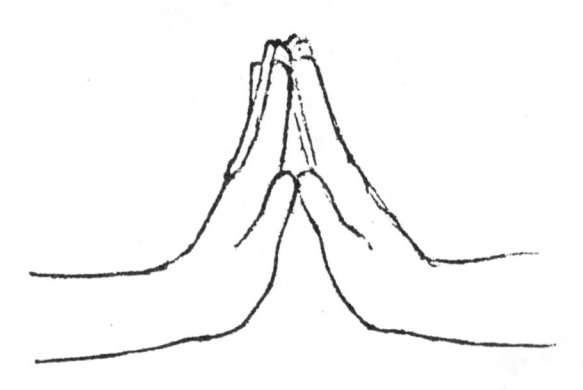

*Introduction*

## 1.4 PRACTICAL THAI MASSAGE

This book is intended to provide you with the basics of Thai massage. The main focus is on practical Thai massage and for that reason the theoretical part of the book has been kept rather short. I have tried to use everyday language and to avoid the use of special medical terminology, thus enabling the layman to easily learn massage techniques which will not only be a source of great pleasure for family and friends but also a contribution to their general well-being.

Thai massage differs radically from 'Swedish Massage' (often called 'Classical Massage') which is the most widespread technique of massage in the West. That kind of massage is very much restricted to working with muscles and soft tissue. Your doctor sends you to a masseur who will knead your muscles for 15 to 30 minutes in an attempt to induce physical and emotional relaxation. There is no doubt but that such relaxing massage plays an important role in a world dominated by haste and stress—but in Thai massage the aspect of muscular relaxation is only a secondary goal. Contrary to Swedish massage, traditional Thai massage does not primarily work with the physical body but rather with the energy body of man. The kneading of muscles which dominates in Swedish massage is absent from Thai massage: energy points are pressed or general pressure is used instead. There is a lot of stretching involved and many exercises might well be described as 'applied Hatha Yoga' or 'applied physical Yoga'. Rather than using the term 'Thai massage', it wouldn't be a bad idea to actually call it 'Yoga massage' since that's what this art essentially is. The tradition is more or less lost in India nowadays, as Ayurvedic massage and Indian Yoga massage have evolved in different directions. But the Yoga background of Thai massage is obvious from all of the beautiful postures used.

Physiotherapy and chiropractice in the West are closer to Thai massage than Swedish massage is, but these techniques also ignore manipulating the energy points and the energy flow of the body: their theoretical foundations are based on the anatomical structure of the body. A search for massage theories and techniques in the West which are more closely parallel to Thai massage brings to mind reflexology, where a workout on energy points is done as well.

The techniques taught in this book are sufficient to enable the beginner to give a full, relaxing whole-body massage, being quite similar to the standard programme of serious massage in Thailand. Such techniques could be termed 'general massage', a kind of massage to be used for massaging more or less anybody. Most masseurs and masseuses in Thailand are trained in this 'general massage'.

In addition, therapeutic massage is practised for the specific treatment of certain diseases. But even in Thailand the extensive knowledge necessary for massage therapy is restricted to experienced specialists. Therapeutic massage is mostly taught through a close and direct personal relationship between student and teacher, and it takes years to learn properly. (See Appendix 3.3 for places which offer long term courses in therapeutic massage.) I have therefore only occasionally given information about the therapeutic use of points, lines and exercises during the course of introducing 'general massage', but in the appendices I do mention how to give basic treatment for headache, backache, and knee pain.

Be responsible in what you are doing! Massage is not a game to be played by irresponsible people. It is a very serious workout on the body and the energy of a fellow human being. This doesn't mean that massage has to be sad-faced and without fun—on the contrary, massage should be joyful for the masseur as well as for the recipient. But careless or inattentive practice of the exercises explained in this book may lead to tension, over-stretching and in extreme cases even to injuries. For such reasons I was initially quite reluctant when I was asked to write this manual of Thai massage. I still highly recommend that beginners should take a practical course in Thai massage with me or another experienced teacher. All novices who do not have that opportunity are asked to carefully follow the methods and advice given for the individual exercises so as to avoid any possible harm.

Especially for a beginner, it is important to slowly develop a feeling for other bodies. Every body is uniquely different, and this means that every massage has to be different, too. The masseur has to 'tune into' the body of each and every patient anew. Stretching exercises may be extremely easy with one person, but if you apply the same stretch to another, less flexible patient, you could do damage. Therefore the masseur has to be extremely careful and sensitive in his approach. While one patient may scream at the slightest thumb pressure, another person won't even feel the same pressure. Generally speaking, pressure should be pleasant but not too soft. Thai massage is by its nature a hard and 'tough' massage, but it most definitely should not be 'torture'.

*Introduction*

## 1.5 TECHNIQUES AND STYLES

The techniques taught in this book give you the structure for a whole-body massage of about 2 to 2 1/2 hours, as long as you don't use repetitions. The beginner will need even a little more time until he gains confidance and experience. Those accustomed to the 15 minute massages of Western-style masseurs may be astonished, but I'm sure your astonishment will soon give way to understanding. You can easily lose track of time entirely while practicing Thai massage.

There are quite a number of massage facilities offering whole-body massages of one hour. These massages either fail to cover the whole body (and so shouldn't be called whole-body massage) or, which is worse, cover the whole body but do so far too quickly. Don't begin your studies with such foolishness. The slower and more intensely you work—without falling into the other extreme of dawdling—the more effective and pleasant is your massage. I don't know a single Thai masseur who is happy giving one hour massages; they are unsatisfactory for masseur and patient alike. From 2 to 2 1/2 hours is regarded as perfect timing for a whole-body massage. This is long enough to treat the whole body, but short enough to maintain concentration. If the massage exceeds 2 1/2 hours it is very difficult for the masseur to maintain full concentration, except for some real masters who can sustain concentration even longer.

For beginners working at home, I suggest that you restrict yourself to one or more sections of the massage if you don't have the time for a full session. It is far better to do one section properly, slowly and with concentration, than to rush slapdash through the whole body.

The structure of the massage I have suggested in this book basically follows the sequence used in traditional Thai massage. The only alteration I have allowed myself is to put the 'face massage in a lying position' at the end of the massage. In traditional Thai massage the face massage is done either at the end of 'the front part of the body in lying position' or at the end of the 'massage in a sitting position'. I prefer to give a long and intensive face massage at the end, in lying position, to ensure deeper and more efficient relaxation.

There are no absolutely fixed rules in Thai massage which restrict the structure and the choice of the exercises. There are hundreds of exercises and virtually every masseur has his own personal style and uses different variations and different sequences. The best masseurs select exercises and sequences according to the needs of the patient.

## The Art of Traditional Thai Massage

Still, there are two reasons why I suggest that beginners follow the structure given in this book. First, the exercises have been selected and structured in such a way that the masseur doesn't have to change position or move about much. Second, the structure is systematic. Easy exercises are done before progressing to more difficult and straining exercises, and thus the body of the recipient is slowly and gradually loosened up.

There are basically two mainstreams of Thai massage in Thailand. They are known as 'Southern Style' and 'Northern Style', and they have developed slightly differently over the centuries. 'Southern Style' is taught at Wat Pho in Bangkok, and 'Northern Style' is taught at the Massage Hospital of the 'Foundation of Shivago Komarpaj' in Chiang Mai. As I practice Northern Style massage, this book is based on that tradition. The techniques and exercises taught in this book and the suggested sequence therefore are only one of many possibilities. Nonetheless, the philosophical foundation for the practice is the same in all styles, in all schools and with all serious masseurs.

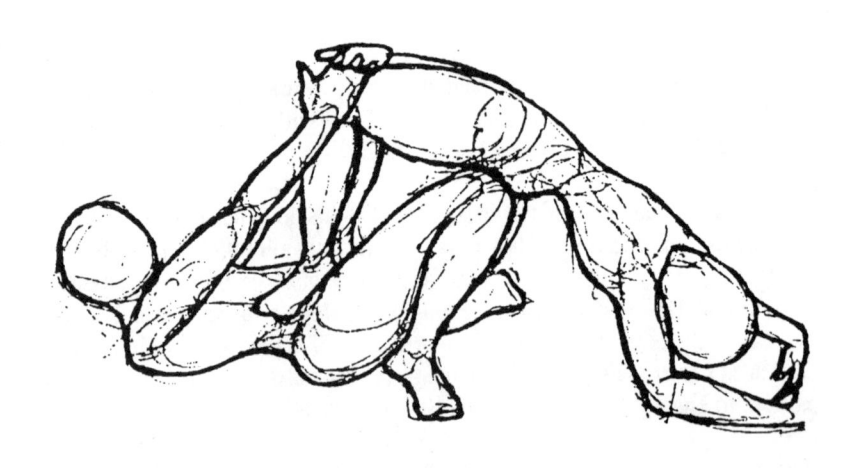

*Introduction*

## 1.6 STATE OF HEALTH OF THE PATIENT

Before starting to give massage it is absolutely essential to enquire about the state of health of your patient:

---

Are there any parts of the body which are especially sensitive or easily damaged?

Is there any acute disease?

Has the patient ever had any operations?

Any heart diseases? High or low blood pressure? Varicose veins? Stomach or intestinal diseases?

Is the patient pregnant?

---

General rules for practical Thai massage are:

Never give massage on bones or on the spine. Don't touch open wounds, infections, blisters and pimples.

In case of heart disease, high blood pressure or varicose veins, never stop the blood flow by blocking the arteries.

No stomach massage should be given in case of serious stomach or intestinal problems. Instead, the emphasis should be on an intensive workout on the energy lines on the back of the body.

The knees are extremely sensitive and can easily be damaged by unskillful pressure. Therefore special care should be observed to avoid excessive strain on the knees.

No hard acupressure should be applied on tired muscles or if the patient is musclebound. There should be no acupressure on lymphatic glands.

Patients with heart conditions should consult their physician before getting a massage. In most cases, doing the lines, light stretching exercises and face massage are possible and beneficial.

Never give stomach massage to pregnant women. After the third month of pregnancy there should be no exercises lying on the stomach and no exercises

13

pregnancy there should be no exercises lying on the stomach and no exercises which involve pressure on the stomach. Only light and easy exercises lying on the back, on the sides, and in a sitting position are allowed. Excellent for pregnant women is a good workout on the energy lines of legs, arms and the back in the sitting position or in the side position, as well as an intensive face massage.

In all cases of patients with chronic and acute diseases, always consult a doctor first and get his approval before massage. As doctors trained in Western medicine tend to be quite conservative when confronted with 'exotic' techniques, my suggestion is to consult doctors who are receptive to alternative methods of treatment: homeopaths, herbal doctors, and Ayurvedic doctors.

Some people react far more sensitively than others to a workout on the energy lines. You may encounter quite a variety of reactions ranging from insomnia to the opposite extreme of heavy weariness, from an incredible mental high to a deep depression. Such diverse responses result from influencing energy streams in the body. The release of negative tension which comes from massage can create feelings of negativity, dragging the recipient down. The unfolding of positive energy streams, on the other hand, may make some people fully awake and agile. Both positive and negative states are only temporary, and so there's no reason to worry. On the contrary, passing through such experiences helps to restore the energy balance of the body.

When giving massage the masseur is acting as an agent for the release of the patient's energies. These energies are channelled through the energy body of the masseur which means that the masseur takes in the energies of his patient. If somebody full of negativity is massaged, this may have a depressing impact on the masseur, making him tired or in extreme cases even sick.

It is therefore important and advisable for the masseur to balance this by meditation or by relaxation exercises right after the massage.

But at least the hands should be washed properly, or better a shower taken, to clean the energy system from the energies of the patient.

The techniques taught in this book foster good health and general well-being— but being able to perform special therapies necessitates sincere study with a good teacher. So don't become presumptuous; this book cannot and was never intended to train you to be a therapist. I sincerely ask you to carefully follow the instructions and warnings given with the exercises.

Once again—seriously sick people need the care of a good doctor. They shouldn't be used as guinea pigs for Thai masseurs-to-be.

*Introduction*

There is no age limit for massage. The massaging of babies by their mothers was probably the oldest form of massage, and even quite elderly people will appreciate your touch as well.

It's very likely that massage is the oldest method of all medical therapies in the history of mankind—far older than all recorded history. People were touching, rubbing and caressing each other both because it felt good and because it helped to heal sickness and to relieve pain. This kind of natural massage is still found in the rural areas of many countries; it is widespread in Thailand's villages even today.

Massage is pleasant and wholesome for men and women alike. Women and men can both give and receive massage, but in certain exercises bodily differences between the sexes have to be taken into account and such differences are specially mentioned. Often in this book I have spoken about the "masseur", "he", etc., using masculine terminology that is in no way intended to offend women. For practical purposes I have surrendered to the patriarchic character of European languages.

Clearly, massage is invaluable for aiding health and well-being. But massage can only be a drop in the ocean so long as one's lifestyle is not based on total health-consciousness. In combination with healthy and nutritious food and a healthy way of life, Thai massage will give you fitness as well as bodily comfort and ease for many years to come.

How often should one get a massage? There are actually no rules or restrictions on frequency. One massage a week is perfectly fine for a whole-body massage. Even every two days is great. And in the case of enthusiasts who like to practice more often, there is no harm in that either.

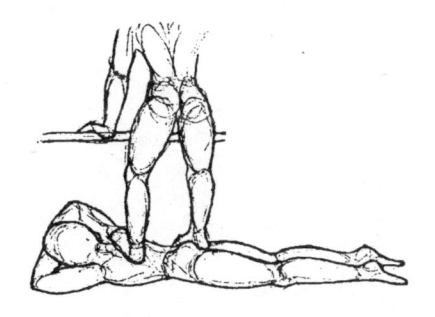

## 1.7 HOW TO LEARN?

You need at least two persons for learning massage. The course outlined in this book is ideal for couples as well as for small groups of people. It is actually helpful to work on different individuals in order to develop a feeling for the variations of bodies. But that doesn't mean that couples won't be able to successfully learn Thai massage.

Create a pleasant atmosphere. Relaxing music and incense sticks are not really essential but they can help to prepare a convivial atmosphere. And a good atmosphere is equally important for furthering the process of learning as well as for aiding the relaxing effect of the massage. Thai massage doesn't use oils except for certain therapies. (For pressure point massage, oil is not useful since it makes the skin slippery.) But it's not such a bad idea to use some good perfume (preferably a floral essence) at the end of the massage to adorn the body of the patient. Take your time while learning and practicing, and make an effort to develop the necessary feeling for each and every section. Don't skip any part but follow the proposed structure systematically. Proceed to the next chapter only when you feel safe and confident about what you have learned so far.

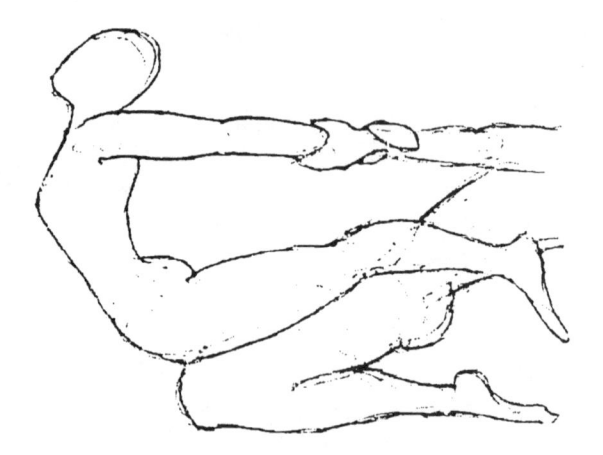

*Introduction*

## 1.8 THE RULES OF A GOOD THAI MASSEUR (AS TAUGHT AT THE MASSAGE HOSPITAL IN CHIANG MAI)

1. Study diligently the techniques and the practice of the massage.

2. Do not practice at public places but at a place suitable for massage.

   *Traditionally a suitable place was a Wat (temple) or a massage hospital. There is no objection to practicing massage at a person's home but to offer your services at, for example, the beach (which is quite common nowadays in Thailand) is regarded as a grave violation of this rule.*

3. Do not hope for any gains, expect neither material profits nor glory or fame.

   *The background of this rule is the concept of massage as a spiritual practice. To give massage is an act of loving-kindness and a meditation—nothing more and nothing less. Massage is not merely a business or a job. Of course the masseur makes his living out of giving massage and must get paid for his work, but neither gaining income nor a desire for honour and praise should be the masseur's motive.*

4. Do not take patients from another masseur.

   *There should not be any competition between masseurs.*

5. Do not boast about your knowledge.

   *Practice what you have learnt and give your best. But be humble and let your massage speak, not your tongue.*

6. Ask for advice and listen to people who know more than you.

7. Bring a good reputation to the "Seven Schools".

   *Well, these "Seven Schools" don't exist in reality. They are meant as a symbol for the whole universe. What this rule really says is: Wherever you work, be aware that you carry responsibility for the reputation of an ancient and revered tradition of healing.*

8. Don't give out certificates in "Basic Thai massage" to a person who is not qualified.

9. Remember and honour daily the roots of the healing massage and it's founder, Jivaka Kumar Bhaccha.

   *Be grateful and do not forget that this is the tradition your work is based on.*

# PART II

# A WHOLE-BODY MASSAGE

*A Whole-body Massage*

## 2.1 THE FRONT PART OF THE BODY

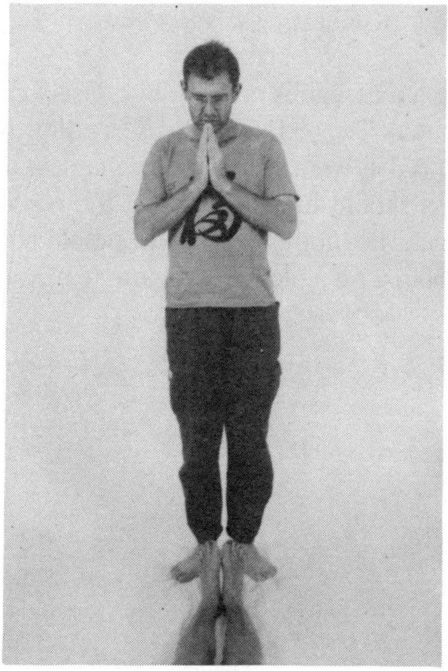

*Illustration 3*

MEDITATIVE PRAYER

Each and every massage should start with a meditative prayer of up to one minute. This is meant to help to centre your mind on the massage and to make it easier to maintain a meditative mood throughout your work. Thai masseurs remember Jivaka Kumar Bhaccha at this moment. They pray that their effort may help to bring freedom from all ailments to their patient. (Illustration 3)

Traditional Thai massage starts with the front part of the body.

Those of you accustomed to Western-style massage may be used to having massage done on a nude body. For cultural reasons this is out of question in Thai massage, which is always done with clothes on. But the recipient should wear light and loose clothing, no jeans or thick sweaters. The masseur's clothing should also be loose so as to enable him to move freely.

In the beginning it's more difficult to massage somebody wearing clothes than to massage someone in the nude since the running of muscles, bones, tendons, etc., is not that obvious. On the other hand the wearing of cloths stimulates sensitivity and reduces the dependence on visual perception, so dominant with most human beings that it may obstruct awareness of the energy flow in the body of the partner. However, what you do at home—massaging with or without clothes—is your own business.

The best place to give a massage is on the floor. Use a comfortable but not overly soft mattress or mat. The recipient can use a pillow if needed. Massage is possible on a double bed as well, as long as the masseur has enough room to move, but the mattress should be hard and not too resilient. Soft beds are impossible for massage. The room temperature should not be too low. For a relaxing massage, a room with a pleasantly warm temperature is essential.

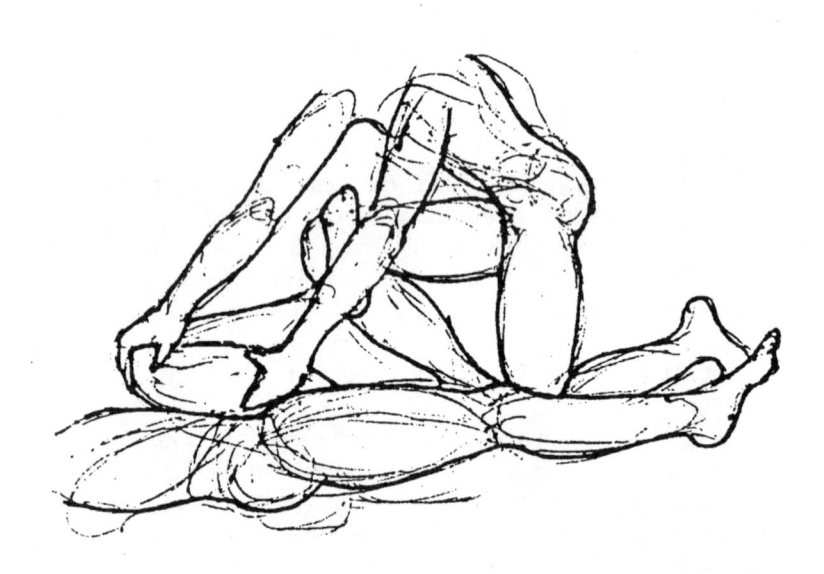

*A Whole-body Massage*

## 2.1.1 FEET

FOOT MASSAGE AND ACUPRESSURE POINTS

The following is a simplified description of some important pressure points and their relationship to the body and its organs.

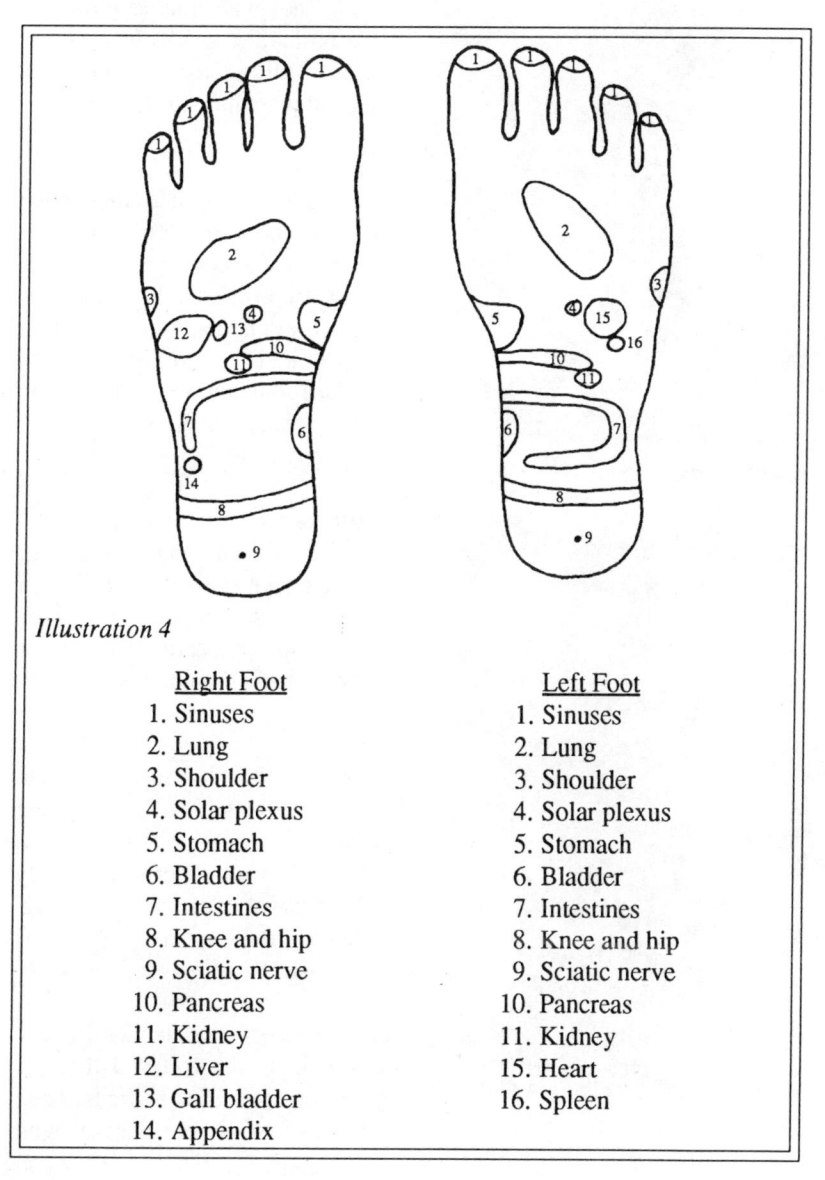

*Illustration 4*

<u>Right Foot</u>
1. Sinuses
2. Lung
3. Shoulder
4. Solar plexus
5. Stomach
6. Bladder
7. Intestines
8. Knee and hip
9. Sciatic nerve
10. Pancreas
11. Kidney
12. Liver
13. Gall bladder
14. Appendix

<u>Left Foot</u>
1. Sinuses
2. Lung
3. Shoulder
4. Solar plexus
5. Stomach
6. Bladder
7. Intestines
8. Knee and hip
9. Sciatic nerve
10. Pancreas
11. Kidney
15. Heart
16. Spleen

23

## WARMING UP AND LOOSENING UP OF THE FEET

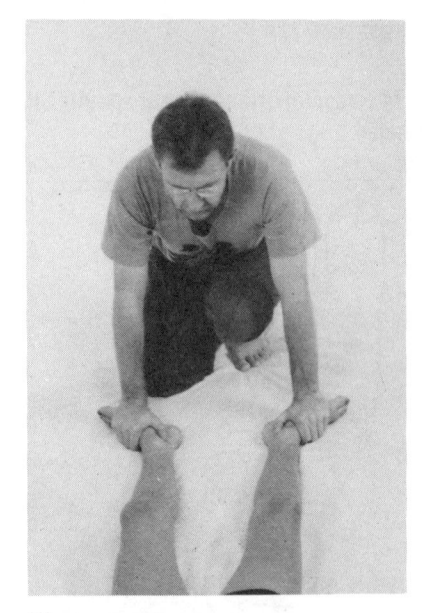

*Illustration 5*

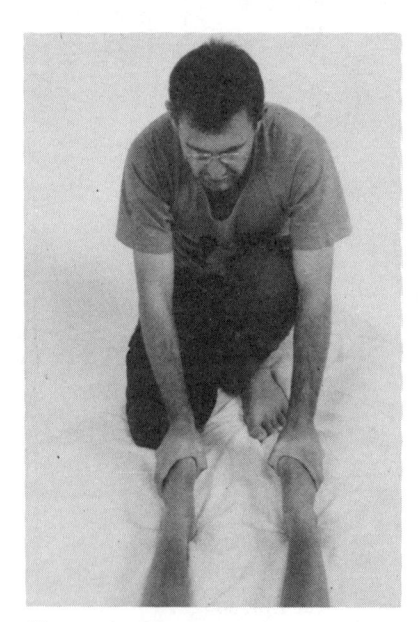

The foot massage starts with warming up and loosening up of the feet. It is important for the masseur to work with straight arms and with body weight, not with muscle power. If these basic rules aren't observed, the masseur will soon pay for it with back pain and premature exhaustion.

Use your palms and push your patient's feet to the side (Illustration 5). Cover the whole sole by moving up and down with your palms. Try to find a body posture that is comfortable for you; one alternative to my posture in Illustration 5 is to kneel on both legs. Use your intuition to find a good posture. That is true for all the coming exercises as well.

**Don't forget:** By now you should have already enquired about your patient's state of health. Also ask if your pressure is getting too painful. Thai massage is a hard and rigourous massage, but it shouldn't be 'torture'.

Observe your 'victim' carefully during the whole massage. Look into his eyes now and then. The blinking of the eyelids and the facial expression will tell you much about how carefully and sensitively you are massaging. Listen to these messages as well as the words spoken by your patient.

Illustration 6 shows another exercise to loosen up the feet and the foot joints. Grasp the feet at the toes and push down with your body weight.

*Illustration 6*

*A Whole-body Massage*

Don't forget to keep your arms straight. Repeat 2-3 times or as often as you like. This is true for all the coming exercises as well.

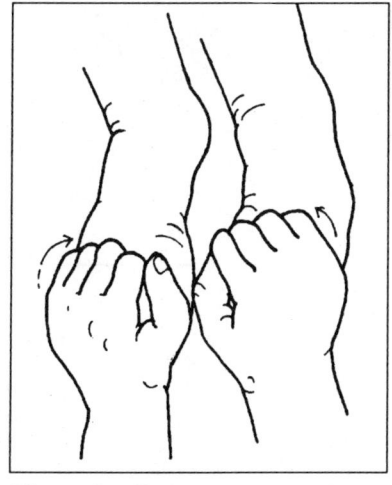

Next grasp around the toes from the front and push with your body weight down towards the patient (Illustration 7).

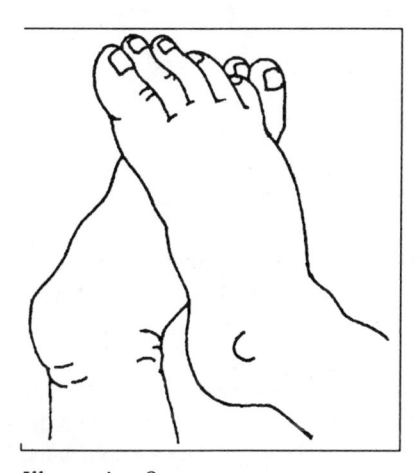

*Illustration 7*

*Illustration 8* 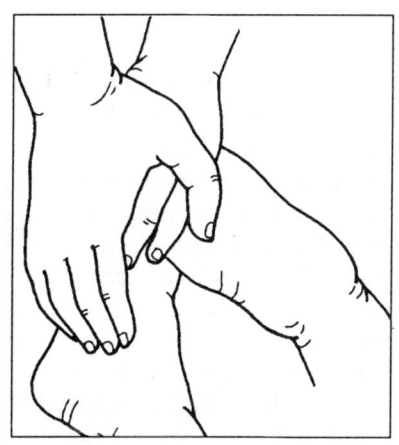   *Illustration 9*

Place one foot on top of the other (Illustration 8) and push down (Illustration 9). This not only loosens up the joints but works as a reflexology massage for the intestines, the kidneys and the stomach. Change feet and repeat the exercise.

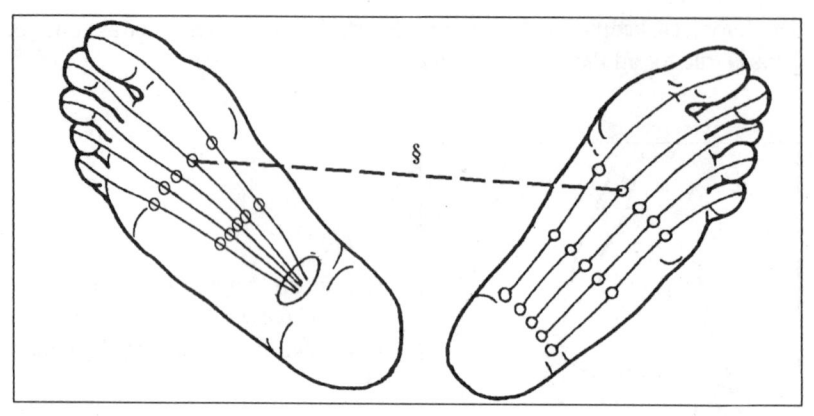

*The Art of Traditional Thai Massage*

*Illustration 10*

## ACUPRESSURE ON THE SOLES OF THE FEET

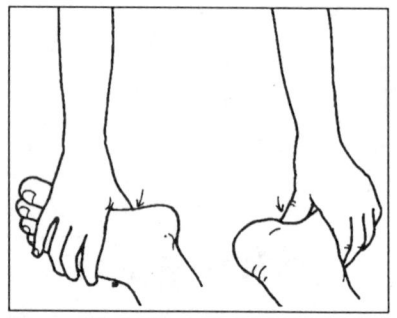

Illustration 10 shows two alternatives for working the soles with thumb pressure (as shown in Illustration 11). Don't forget to keep your arms straight and to use your body weight.

*Illustration 11*

In Illustration 10, left, you start with pressure on one point in the centre of the feet just past the heels. This is a therapy point to counter foot pain and insomnia. Work with thumb pressure along the indicated points towards the toes. You automatically cover several of the acupressure points shown in Illustration 4. There is nothing you can do wrong! Wherever you press you will hit a point beneficial for an organ or a part of the body.

In the front part of the feet, starting with the ball of the foot, don't apply any more thumb pressure since you will hit bone. Do some soft rubbing with the thumbs towards the toes instead. Press the tips of the toes. They are connected with the sinuses. Pay special attention to the point marked §. This is a therapy point for the treatment of shock, sunstroke, and hypertension.

Illustration 10, right, shows a different variation. You don't start from one centre point, but instead you will work in straight lines towards the toes.

## A Whole-body Massage

> So far we have been working parallel on both feet at the same time. Now we proceed with one leg at a time. With men we start with the right foot, with women we start with the left. This usage recalls the Chinese philosophy of Yin and Yang, or the male and female aspect. The left part of the brain is seen as the 'rational' or the 'male' part and it controls the right side of the body. The right part of the brain then is the 'intuitive', the 'female' side and it controls the left side of the body. So with men we start on the male side, with women on the female side. This is true for all the coming exercises as well.

RELAXING OF THE FOOT JOINTS

Lift the foot as in Illustration 12 and move it in large circles to the left and to the right.

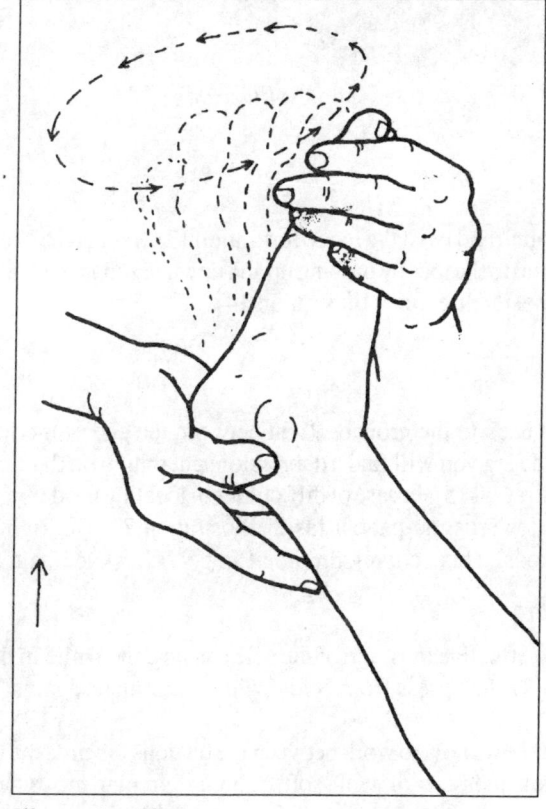

*Illustration 12*

27

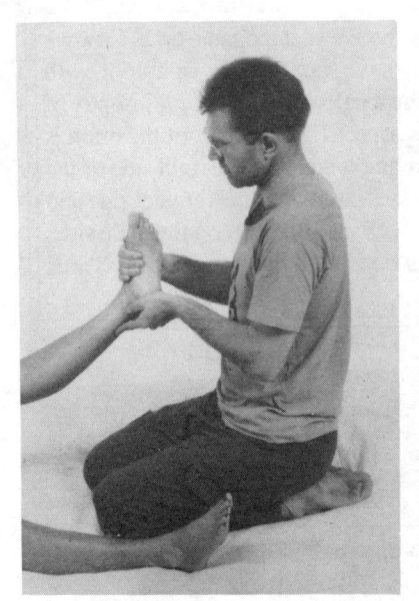

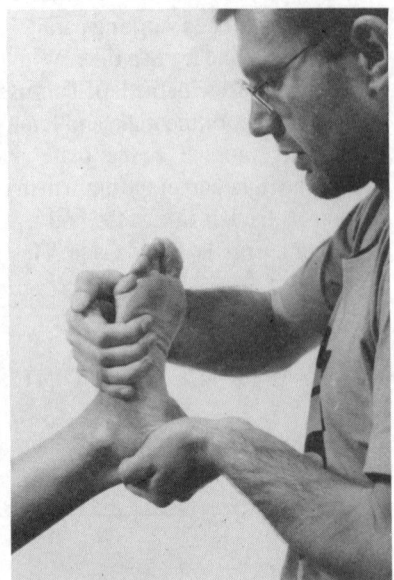

*Illustration 13*  *Illustration 14*

Then grasp around and twist the foot (Illustration 13). Start at the heel and work the whole foot up to the toes by moving up and down. Exchange hands and twist the foot in opposite direction (Illustration 14).

RELAXING THE FEET

Bring the foot back to the ground. Right between the end of the foot and the beginning of the leg you will find a depression; put thumb on thumb and apply pressure (Illustration 15). In case of difficulties in locating the depression, push the foot back towards the patient (as in Illustration 7). The right spot then becomes obvious. This acupressure point is good for knee pain as well as headache.

A pleasant and effective massage of the sole can be done while in the position of Illustration 15. Just press from below with your fingers against the sole.

Illustration 16 shows how to work between the tendons towards the toes, either by using thumb pressure or with soft, rubbing circular movements of the thumbs.

## A Whole-body Massage

*Illustration 15*

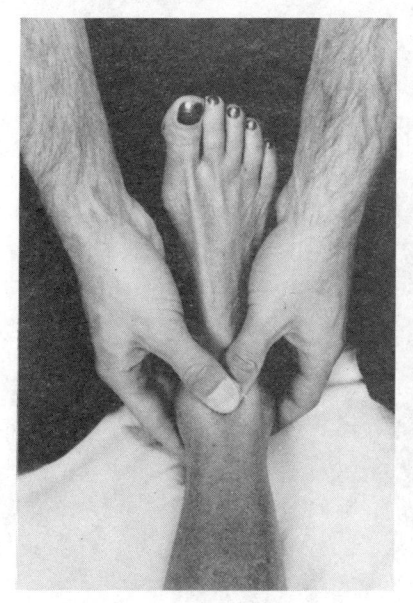

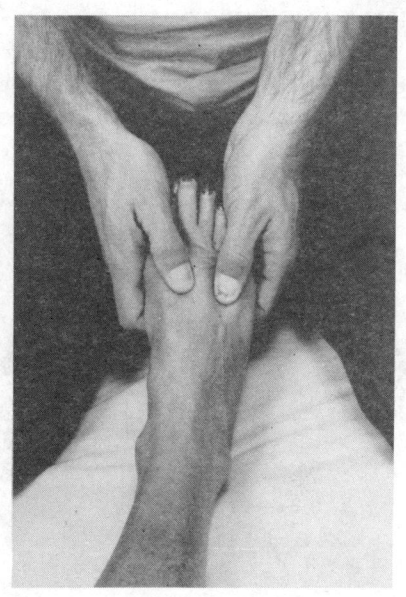

*Illustration 16*

### CRACKING THE TOES

Crack one toe after the other with a gentle but determined tug (Illustration 17). You may need some practice to crack the toes properly so that you can hear them 'crack'. This exercise relaxes the toe joints. Every now and then some of the toes—or even all of them—won't crack at all. In such cases, don't bother about it too much. Don't try to attain the goal by pulling extra hard or pulling several times. And don't crack the toes more than once during one massage.

After you've finished, change to the other foot and repeat all the exercises described so far.

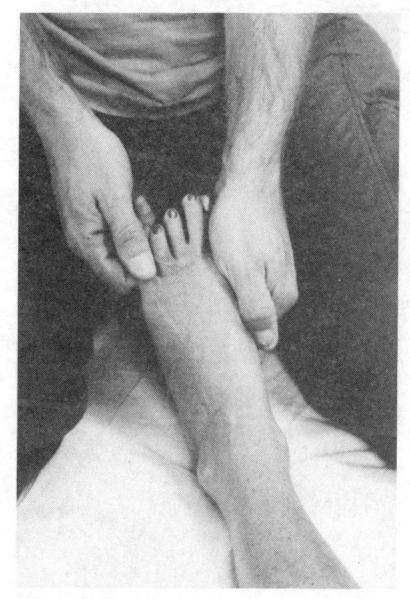

*Illustration 17*

29

## FINISHING THE FOOT MASSAGE

Finish the foot massage by pressing the tips of the toes (Illustration 18) and repeat the exercises introduced in the beginning of this chapter, "Warming up and loosening up of the feet".

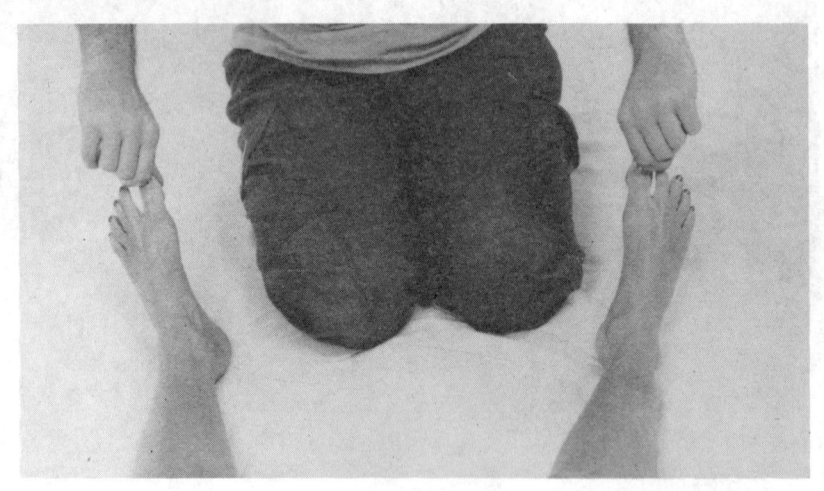

*Illustration 18*

*A Whole-body Massage*

## 2.1.2 ENERGY LINES ON THE LEGS

THE ENERGY LINES ON THE INSIDE OF THE LEGS

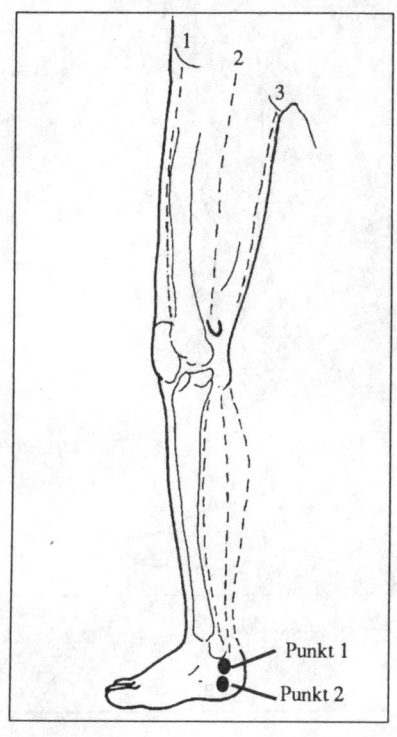

Illustration 19 shows the running of the energy lines on the inside of the legs. As these are not anatomical lines, the representation given here can only be a rough guide line. Try to develop a feeling for the lines. Be open and trust your feelings.

**Line 1** on the lower leg runs just below the shin bone (tibia). On the thigh the line starts on the extension of the outmost edge of the patella and moves straight up towards the groin.

**Line 2** on the lower leg can be located by the depression to the side of the ankle bone (between the ankle bone protrusion and the Achilles tendon). On the thigh there is another depression at the side of the knee which indicates the start of the line which then moves straight up to the groin.

*Illustration 19*

**Line 3** on the lower leg runs along the Achilles tendon, along the back of the calf. On the thigh you can feel a tendon and you work above the tendon towards the groin.

**Point 1** lies directly below the ankle. This point is very painful. It is connected with the sexual organs and is a therapy point for menstruation problems, impotence, etc.

For a relaxing massage **Point 2** is pressed instead as it is much less painful and influences Point 1 indirectly.

**Caution**: In case of pregnancy pressure on both these points is prohibited!

## THE ENERGY LINES ON THE OUTSIDE OF THE LEGS

Illustration 20 shows energy lines on the outside of the legs. Just as on the inside of the leg, we work three lines on the outside of the leg. But the third line is easier to treat in the side position and will therefore be dealt with later.

**Line 1** on the lower leg runs directly below the shin bone. On the thigh the line starts at the outmost edge of the patella and moves towards the hip.

**Line 2** on the lower leg starts at the upper side of the ankle above the outer ankle bone protrusion (malleolus externus), on top of the fibula bone.

On the thigh the start of the line can be located by a depression to the side of the knee.

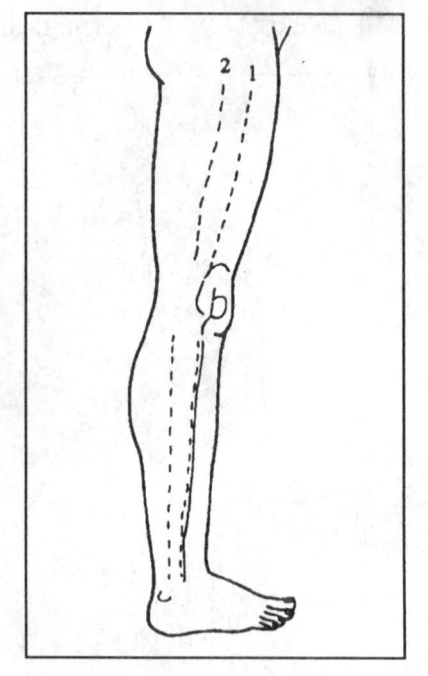

*Illustration 20*

## HOW TO WORK THE ENERGY LINES

### 1. Palming

Apply pressure along the lines with the palms of your hands. Work with straight arms and shift your body weight from one side to the other (Illustration 21).

Palming is relaxing and pleasant. Take your time. Play up and down the legs with rhythmic movements as often as you like but at least two or three times.

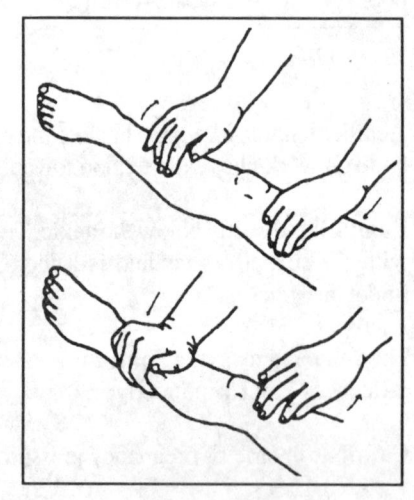

*Illustration 21*

*A Whole-body Massage*

## 2. Thumbing

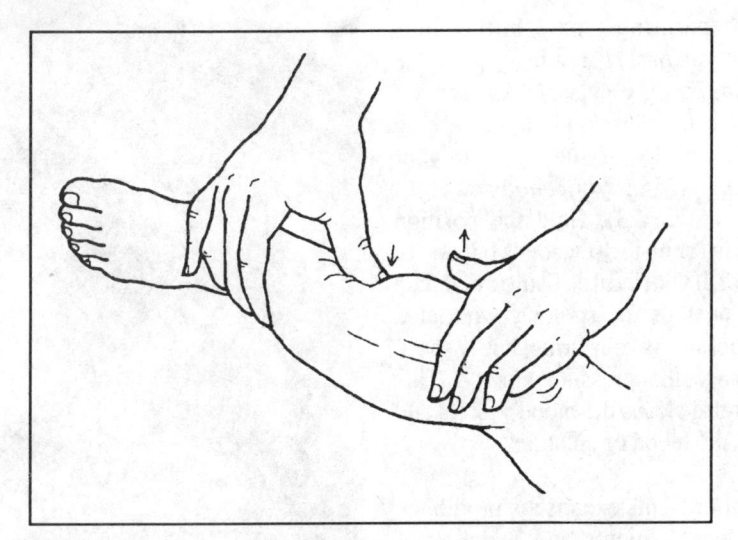

*Illustration 22*

Work along the lines with one thumb pressing, sustaining the pressure a little while (Illustration 22). The second thumb is placed next to the first one. While the second thumb increases the pressure, the first thumb is slowly lifted. In this way work up and down all the lines.

Line 3 on the lower inside leg is worked either by pressing from above on the Achilles tendon or you press the tendon from below.

Work from one side. First palming and thumbing the inside of one leg, then the outside of the other leg. When dealing with the outside lines it may be necessary to turn the leg a little to enable you to reach the lines. Change to the other side and press the inside lines of one leg first, then the outside lines of the other leg.

Concentrate and work slowly but in a flowing style.

**Caution**: Leave the knees alone! The knees are very sensitive and are easily damaged by unskillful pressure.

## STOPPING THE BLOOD FLOW TO THE LEGS

Do palming on both legs simultaneously, moving up to the groin. Feel the pulse. When you are sure of the pulse on both sides, stop the blood flow to the legs with your palms, using your body weight (Illustration 23). Hold the position firmly for up to 50 seconds but do not shake. If you find it difficult to maintain the posture for so long without a trembling in your arms, cut it short. Release the pressure slowly. This exercise cleans the blood vessels and aids the blood circulation.

**Caution**: This exercise is prohibited for heart patients and in cases of hypertension and varicose veins.

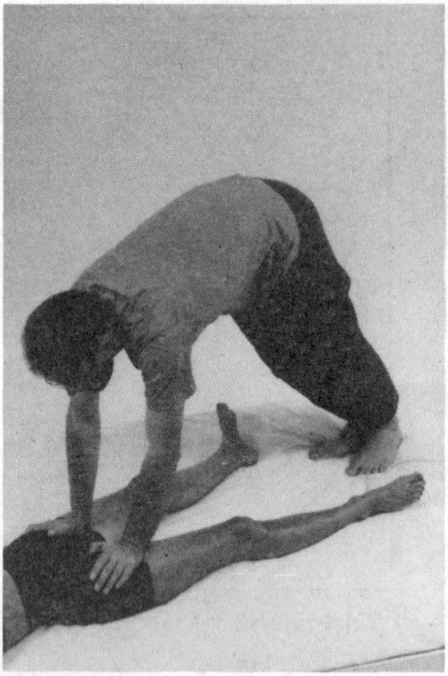

*Illustration 23*

*A Whole-body Massage*

## 2.1.3 EXERCISES WITH ONE LEG

ONE LEG POSITIONS

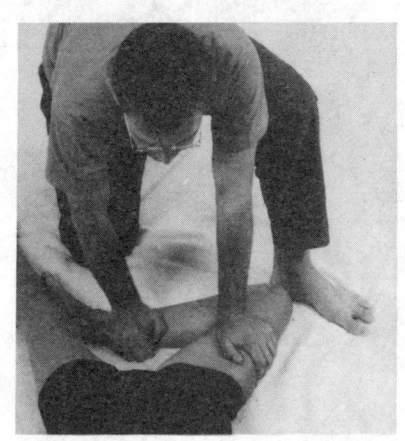

*Illustration 24*

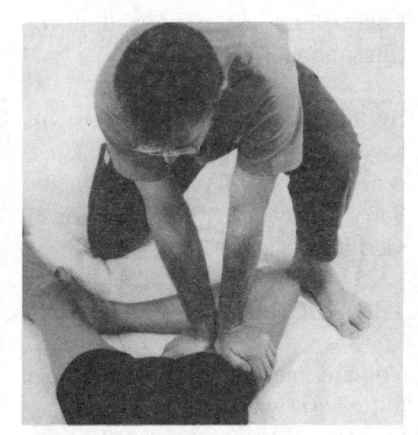

*Illustration 25*

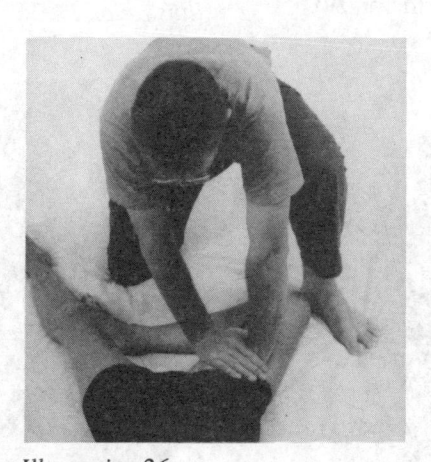

*Illustration 26*

Start with palming on one leg (men, right leg; women, left leg). The leg of the patient is bent. Examples of different techniques of palming are depicted in Illustrations 24, 25 and 26. Don't be shy, use your imagination.

Work the whole leg but stay away from the knee.

## THE CALF

Put up the patient's bent leg and fix the toes with your toes. Separate the calf muscle in the centre with your fingers and move up and down (Illustration 27).

By this point at the latest you will have discovered that giving a massage is not possible with long fingernails. Sorry, but you'll probably have to sacrifice the nails ...

## THE THIGH

You are kneeling, and the foot and lower leg of your patient are between your legs. Work the whole thigh with your palms (Illustration 28) and with your thumbs (Illustration 29).

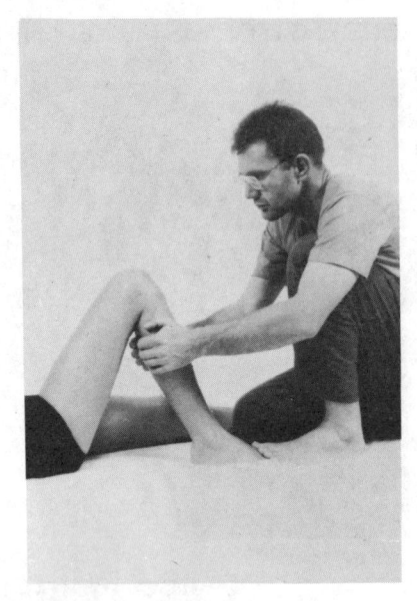

*Illustration 27*

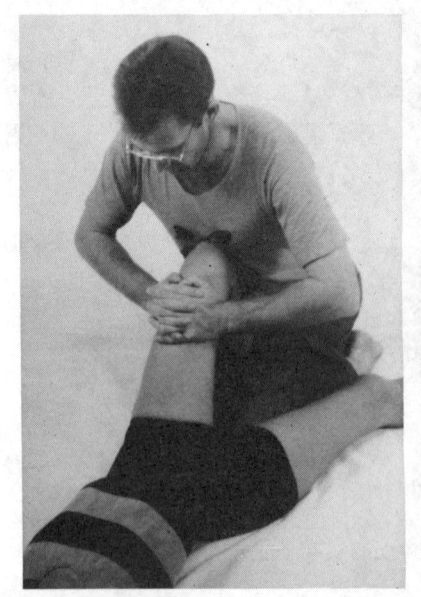

*Illustration 28*

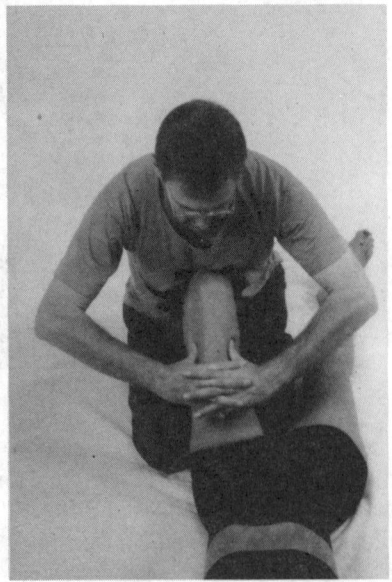

*Illustration 29*

## A Whole-body Massage

At first your thumbs might be weak and thumbing may be quite a hard and difficult exercise to do. To get your thumbs strong enough will take time, probably a couple of months. Exercise your thumbs by kneading a small ball of wax whenever you have nothing else to do (while watching TV, going for a walk, etc.).

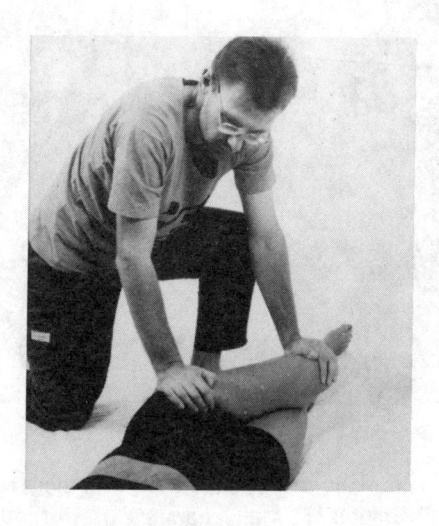

*Illustration 30*

Push the bent leg to the side so that it rests on the straight leg. Fix the knee with one hand. Do palming on the whole thigh (Illustration 30).

It is not easy, but very effective, to do thumbing on the first and the second outside line of the thigh. Give it a try.

This is also a good position for doing the third outside line, which will be introduced later (see Illustration 68).

After this exercise it might be a good idea to stretch out and relax the leg by repeatedly bending and stretching it. In any of the postures that follow you may do this kind of relaxing movement whenever you feel that there was a lot of strain on the patient's leg.

37

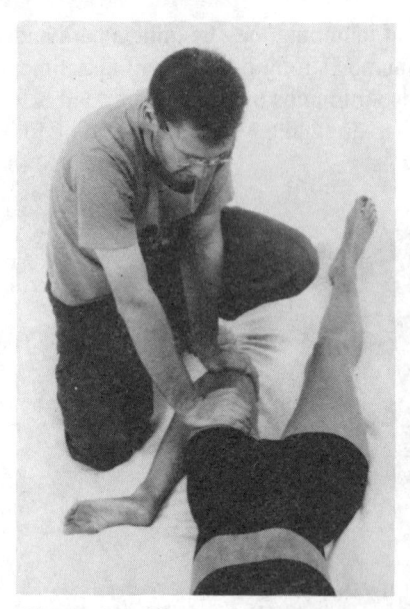

*Illustration 31* 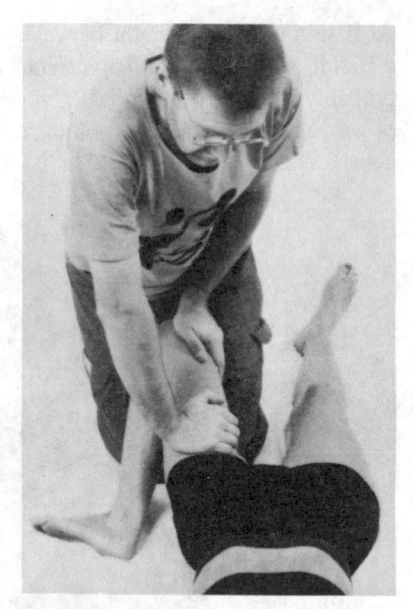  *Illustration 32*

For most Asians it is normally easy to put the leg with the lower leg bent right down to the floor (Illustration 31). Many 'Farangs' (*farang* is the Thai word for any foreigner of European descent) experience a lot of difficulties in having this done to them, being spoiled by sitting on chairs. (Chairs, by the way, are responsible for quite a number of problems with stiffness and tension.)

Don't force your patient into the position of Illustration 31. If it is impossible to place the leg on the ground comfortably, use the 'Farang Aid' depicted in Illustration 32 as an alternative. In that position you are able to arrange the patient's position precisely to suit his flexibility by simply moving his leg higher or lower on both your thighs.

One hand is holding the knee in place, while the other hand is palming the whole thigh.

STRETCHED LEG, STRETCHED TENDON

Put the stretched leg on your lower leg near the foot joint and stretch it out as far as comfortably possible (Illustration 33 and 34). In case the patient's other leg lifts off the ground you may hold it with your lower leg as depicted in Illustration 33.

## A Whole-body Massage

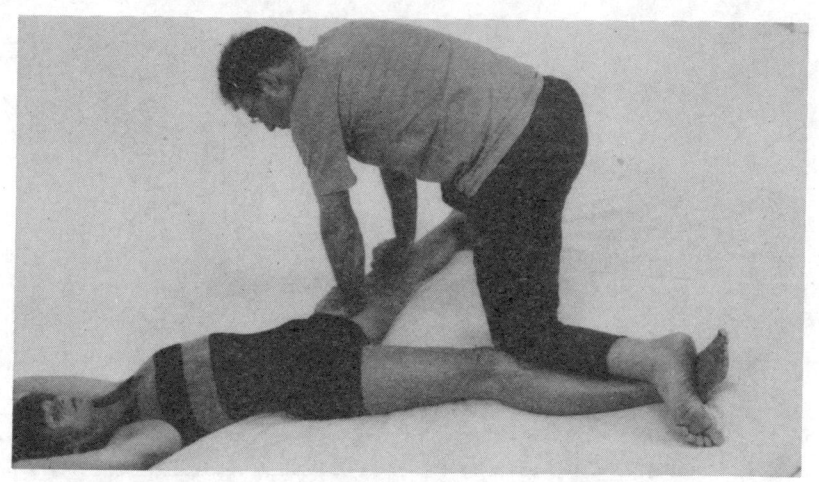

*Illustration 33*

To prevent straining the knee put one hand on the knee but without pressure, just stabilizing it. (See the positioning of the right hand in Illustration 34.) In this exercise it is important to work the stretched tendon of the thigh, where the third inside line of the leg runs. (See the positioning of my left hand on Illustrations 33 and 34.) Do palming along the whole thigh. Skip the lower leg as working on it in this position may apply too much pressure on the knee. It is possible, but not absolutely essential, to do palming and thumbing on the second and first inside line on the thigh as well.

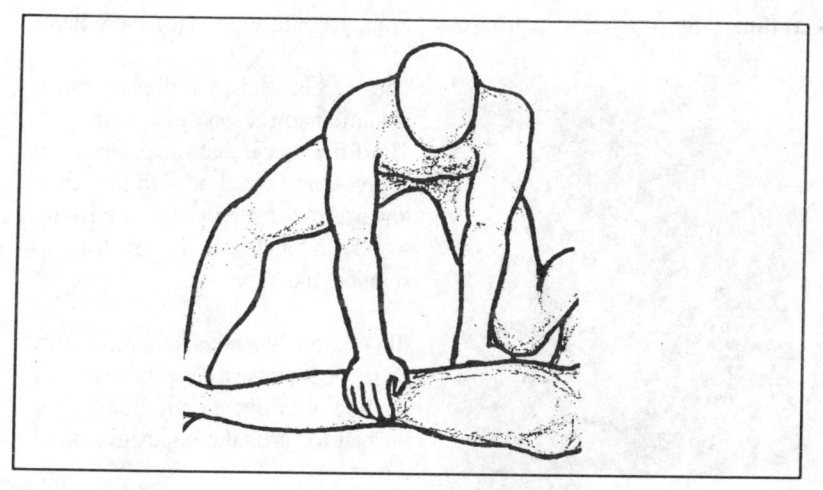

*Illustration 34*

*The Art of Traditional Thai Massage*

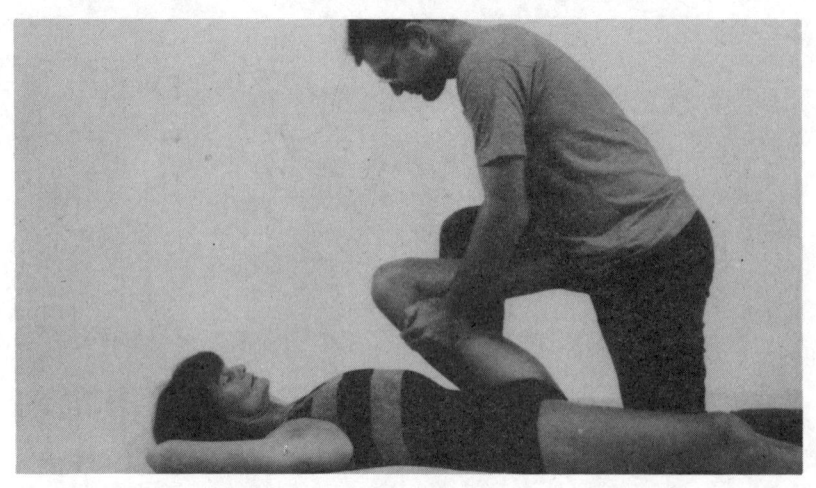

*Illustration 35*

Place the patient's foot on your groin area. With your body weight push his leg towards the chest (Illustration 35). Release the pressure, put your hands one hand span lower on the thigh, and then repeat. In the third repetition move your hands yet another hand span lower.

This exercise not only stretches the muscles and tendons of the thigh and opens up the groin and hip area but it is also excellent for indigestion and a bloated abdomen.

**Caution:** Skip this exercise in case of hernia. It could aggravate the problem.

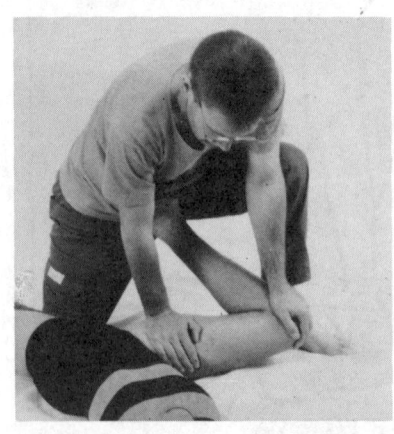

The exercise shown in Illustration 36 is similar to the one just explained. The difference is that you push the leg away from the body rather than towards the chest. Instead of pushing with both hands you use one hand to stabilise the knee.

Illustration 37 shows the third in this series of exercises. Here the leg is not pushed straight down but rather pushed towards the opposite side of the chest.

*Illustration 36*

40

## A Whole-body Massage

**Caution:** Often even the slightest pressure can be extremely painful for the patient.

From the position in Illustration 37 just let yourself fall back on your buttocks. Entwine the foot and leg of the bent leg as shown in Illustration 38 and then grasp around the heel with your hand. Pull back on the heel using your body weight and 'walk' up and down the thigh with your other leg. Whenever you stretch that leg, pull back with your body; whenever you release the pressure, release the pull as well. The nearer you sit to the patient, the heavier the pressure you apply when you stretch your leg. Another possibility for controlling the pressure is to use your heel (for hard pressure) or the ball of your foot (for soft pressure).

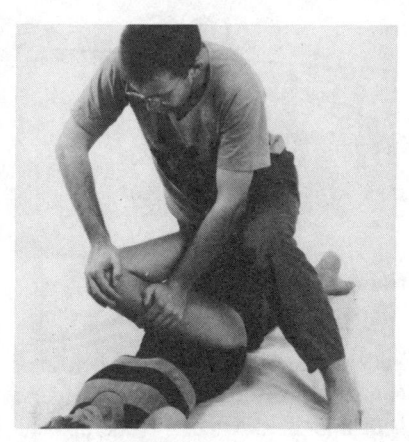

*Illustration 37*

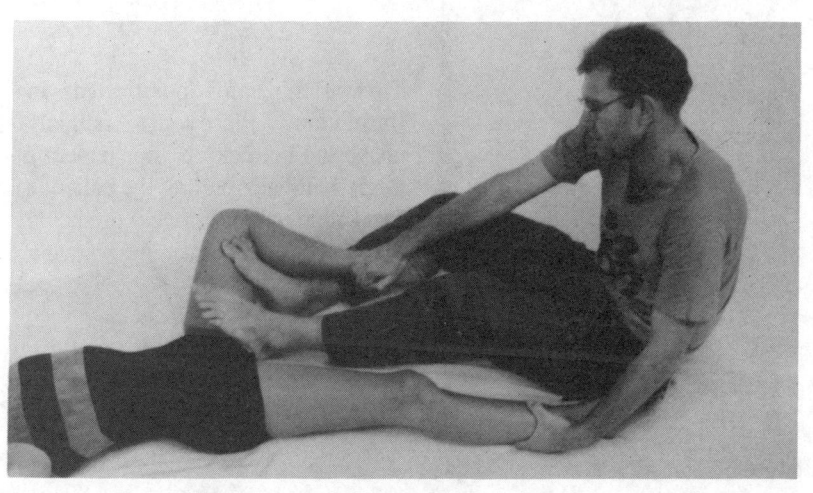

*Illustration 38*

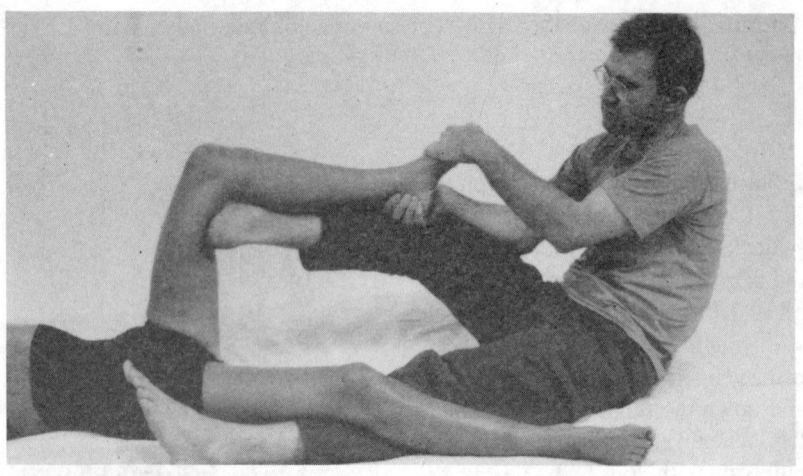

*Illustration 39*

Put your straight leg either below or above the straight leg of the patient (Illustration 39). The bent leg, which is lifted up, is grasped by the foot at the heel and at the toes. Walk up and down the thigh while pulling back simultaneously on the foot using your body weight.

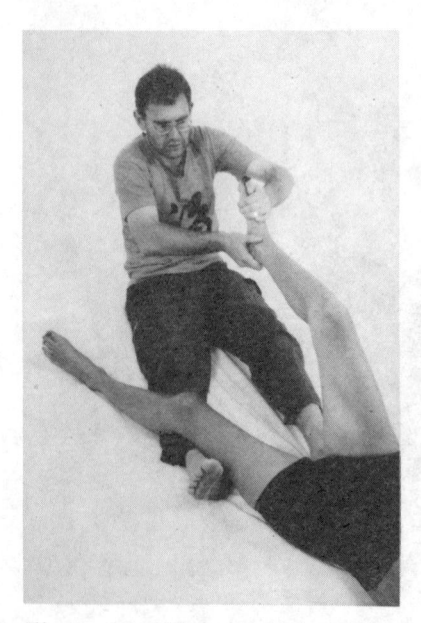

This is the same position as in Illustration 39. Place your foot slightly above the buttock on your patient's thigh. Fall back pulling the patient's foot and stretching his leg. You should feel the bottom bone rolling over your toes (Illustration 40).

Sometimes this exercise is painful for the toes. Feel free to skip it then.

*Illustration 40*

## A Whole-body Massage

Move towards the patient and put his bent leg across your leg at the foot joint (Illustration 41). Grasp and work with your fingers the first and the second outside lines of the thigh.

**Variation**   Do the same exercise but bring your legs together and put the patient's bent leg across both of your legs. This may be an easier position for you; try it and find out for yourself.

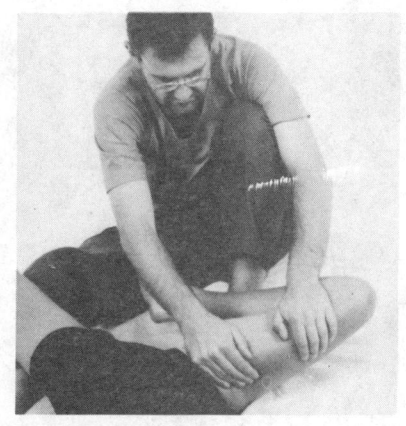

*Illustration 41*

Get up and hold the patient's slightly bent leg at the heel. Do palming along the thigh using your body weight (you cover the third outside line of the thigh). Whenever you give pressure with your palms, push the leg a bit inwards towards the sternum and at the same time towards the head (Illustration 42).

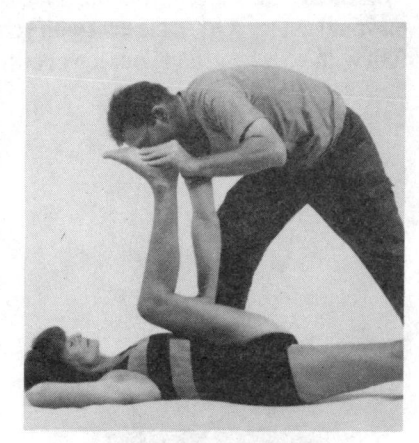

*Illustration 42*

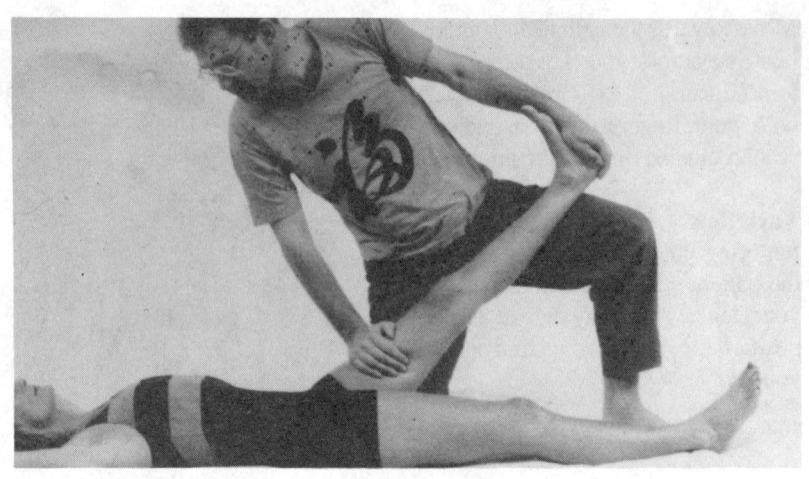

*Illustration 43*

STRETCHING OF THE STRAIGHT LEG

You kneel with one leg, your other leg is bent. Place your patient's straight leg on your bent leg. Grasp his heel with your hand and cover the whole sole of the foot with your hand and your lower arm. Your other hand works up and down the thigh while with every application of pressure you push down the foot with your lower arm (Illustration 43)

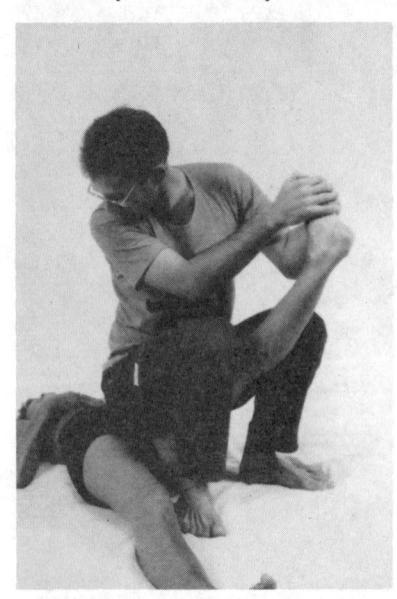

**Caution:** While palming take care to stay quite a distance away from the knee to avoid damaging it. Restrict your palming to the thigh only. In any case, the pressure with your palms is less important than the pushing of the foot with your lower arm.

The exercise depicted in Illustration 44 is similar but more strain-inducing than the one explained with Illustration 43. It is especially effective for the lower leg but use it only with flexible people.

*Illustration 44*

## A Whole-body Massage

Fix the thigh with your buttocks (avoid too much pressure, so don't actually sit on your patient's leg). Hold the foot with both hands at the ball of the foot and the toes. Pull the foot upwards and at the same time pull down on the toes.

### EKAPADA UTTANAPADA ASANA

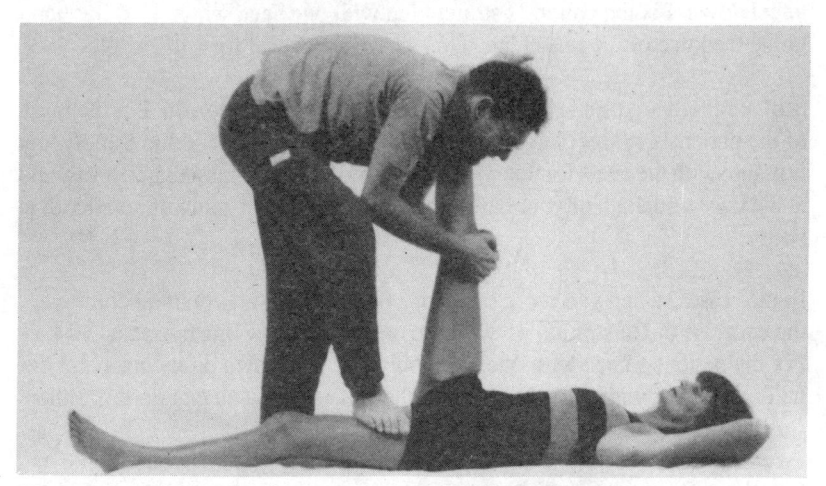

*Illustration 45*

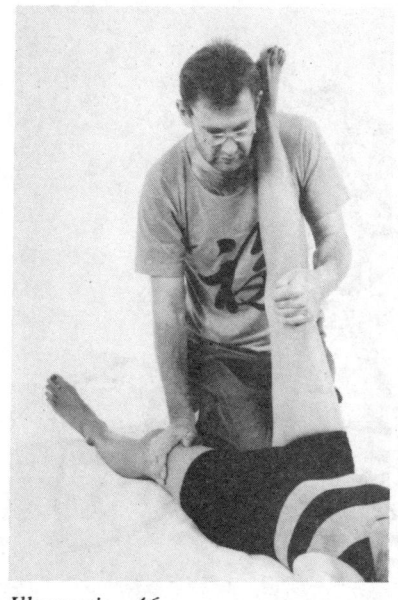

*Illustration 46*

A rigorous but very effective stretching exercise with the Sanskrit name of Ekapada Uttanapada Asana is depicted in Illustration 45 and 46. You are standing. The patient's straight, elevated leg is placed on your shoulder. Use your foot to fix the thigh (but don't apply pressure, only fix the leg!). Grasp around the knee with both hands. Push with your body slowly towards the head of the patient (Illustration 45).

With a very limber person it would be possible to bring the leg right to the ground behind the head. With a stiff patient you may not even be able to reach as far as is shown in Illustration 45. Stretch to the limit and then hold the position for some seconds.

*The Art of Traditional Thai Massage*

**Caution:** Don't overdo it. Don't over-stretch. Let your patient tell you when you've reached the limit until you have developed feeling for it.

Illustration 46 shows a variation which might be easier to do, depending on you and your patient's size, weight and flexibility. Experiment. Instead of standing, kneel down. Fix the patient's straight leg with one hand while the other hand holds the knee of the raised leg. This variation is ideal for stiff people.

Still another variation is based on the position in Illustration 46. Fix the thigh of the patient's straight leg on the floor with your knee—but don't apply any pressure with the knee, for this would be far too painful! The elevated leg is held at the knee with both of your hands. Try this variation on patients smaller than you.

In rare cases, when you work on a very flexible patient, you may combine the exercise of Illustration 45 with the one depicted in Illustrations 43/44. Fix the patient's knee with one hand only and pull down on the toes and the ball of the foot with the other hand at the same time. You can do this either from the standing, or from the kneeling position.

**Caution:** This technique intensifies the effect of the exercise tremendously. It might be very painful, if you are not careful enough.

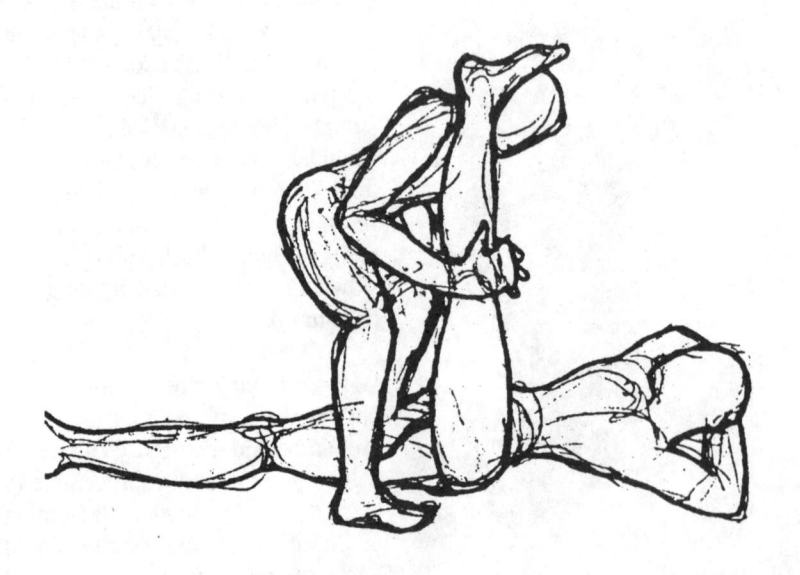

## A Whole-body Massage

## SPINAL TWIST

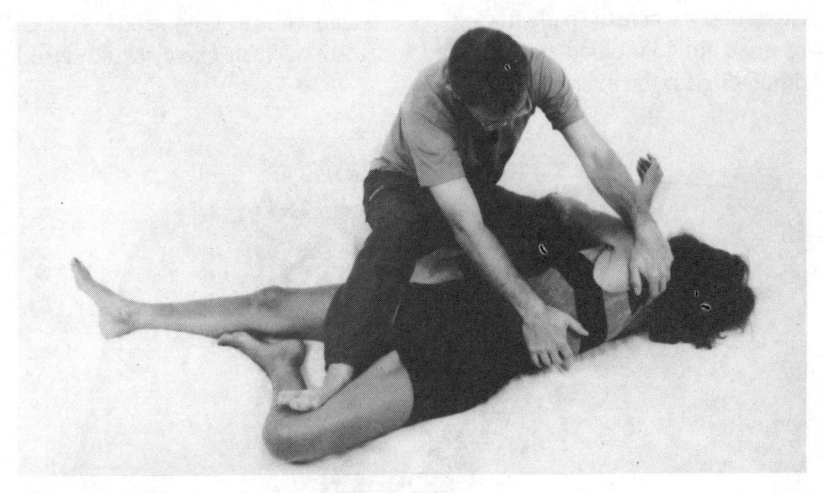

*Illustration 47*

An excellent exercise for the spine is shown in Illustration 47. Sit with one leg bent at the side of the patient.

The patient's bent leg is fixed with your other leg. One of the patient's arms rests on the floor. Grasp his other arm with both hands (one hand on the lower arm, one hand on the upper arm) and then slowly and gently pull the body to the side, lifting the patient's shoulder off the ground. Then grasp over as depicted in Illustration 47 and work with your fingers and hands up and down the back.

You may hear some cracking of the spine. Well, that's perfectly fine since the exercise helps correct spinal problems.

You have now completed the exercises with one leg. Repeat the whole sequence with the other leg.

## 2.1.4 EXERCISES WITH TWO LEGS

All exercises where the patient's legs are elevated while he is lying on his back are good for low blood pressure and indigestion. Such exercises are also stimulating for the internal organs.

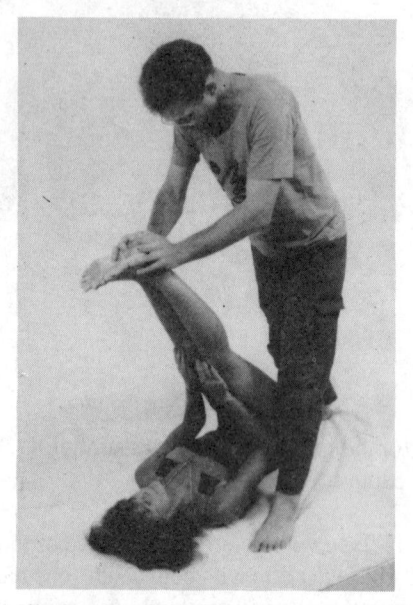

*Illustration 48*

### THE PLOUGH

Raise the legs and ask the patient to put his hands on his knees to stabilise the posture shown in Illustration 48. Then push the legs towards the head, first a little bit, then a little bit more and finally as far as you can comfortably push, depending on the flexibility of the patient. With very limber people you may bring the straight legs right to the floor behind the head. (This is the Yoga posture of Hala-Asana or 'The Plough').

**Caution:** The Plough is prohibited for women during menstruation. I don't recommend this exercise in cases of high blood pressure or heart diseases either.

*A Whole-body Massage*

Stand with your feet next to the patient's armpits. Bring the patient's feet together and push them down to the floor behind his head. Give way with your knees while you push so not to obstruct the movement (Illustration 49). This is the Yoga posture of Karna Peeda Asana.

**Caution**: With many people it will be impossible to bring the feet to the floor. Don't force it.

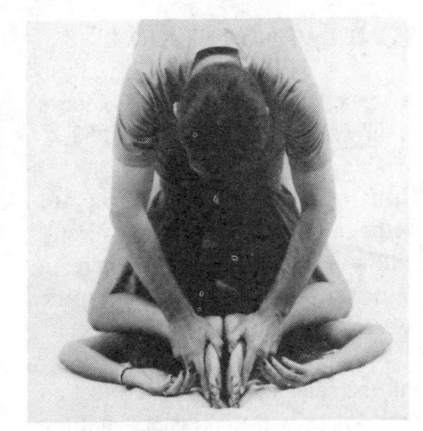

*Illustration 49*

Move your feet back half a step and push the patient's legs straight down towards the nose (Illustration 50). With very flexible people you can touch the nose with the feet. This is the Yoga posture of Baddha Kona Asana.

**Caution**: Skip the exercises depicted in Illustration 49 and 50 in cases of high blood pressure, heart disease and during menstruation.

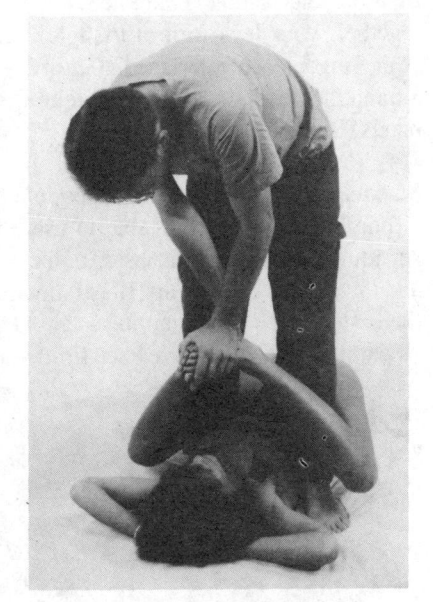

*Illustration 50*

*The Art of Traditional Thai Massage*

## STIMULATING THE KIDNEYS

An excellent exercise for the kidneys is shown in Illustration 51 and 52.

**Caution**: This exercise is not without danger. Therefore strictly follow the explanations given here. In case of any doubt, you should skip the exercise.

Put the soles of the patient's feet on your knees with the instep—not the heel, and not the ball of the foot!—right on your patella. Your knees are together, your legs form a triangle, your fingers are interlaced. Grasp around the patient's thighs with your hands (Illustration 51).

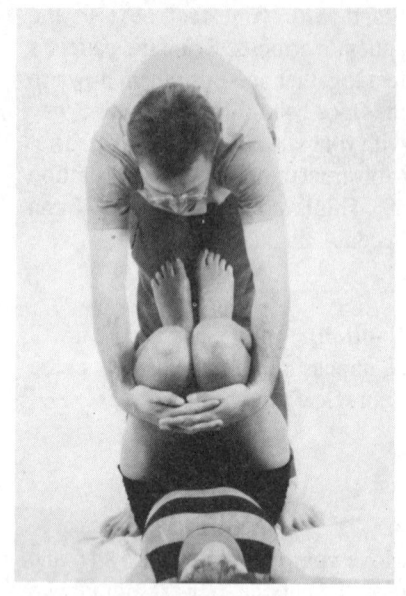

*Illustration 51*

Stand as near to the patient as possible (i.e., without losing your balance or falling back) so as to be able to use leverage. Go down on your knees—squatting, not sitting! The instep of the patient's feet rolls over your knee caps and the patient is lifted up (Illustration 52). Your posture must be stable and there should be no trembling—thus the triangular position of the legs is essential. Your hands have to be firmly interlaced and your grip must be tight.

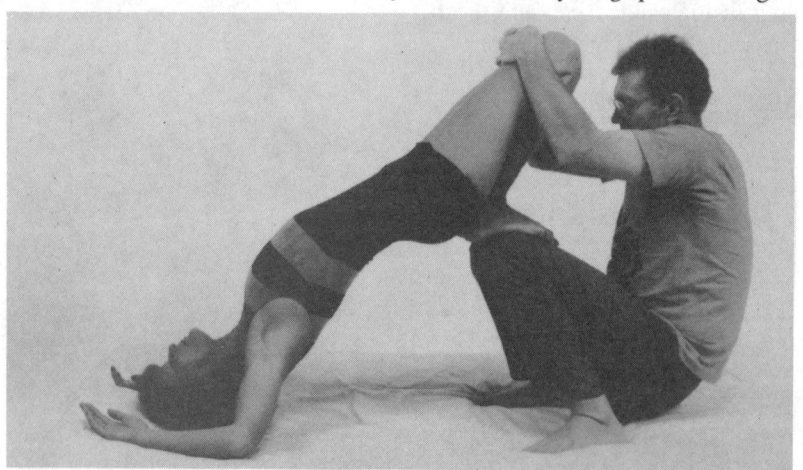

*Illustration 52*

## A Whole-body Massage

Come out of the kneeling position slowly after having held the posture for some seconds. Bring your patient's torso gently back to the floor.

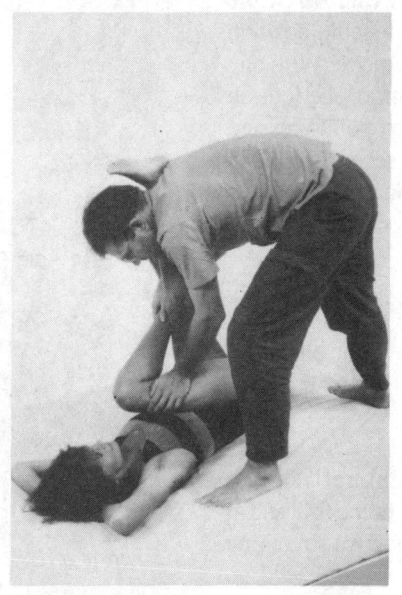

*Illustration 53*

Then, one of the patient's legs is bent and placed on the thigh above the knee (Illustration 53). Put the straight leg on your shoulder. One hand grasps the patient's foot joint and ankle, while the other hand palms the thigh of the bent leg (working on the second and third outside lines on the thigh). Push the bent leg towards the centre of the body, the sternum.

**Caution:** Don't force this exercise (or the following one) on stiff people or people with knee problems.

## 'THE SPANISH INQUISITION'

Entwine the bent leg with your leg (Illustration 54). Take care to have the patient in a firm and stable position where his legs can't move. With one hand hold the dorsum of the foot on the straight leg and give point-pressure with your elbow on several points in the centre of the foot. Press, hold for some seconds, and then release slowly.

In case your patient is much bigger than you it might be difficult to reach the footsole with the elbow. You can then work with your thumbs instead.

This is an excellent reflexology massage for the sole of the foot and at the same time an effective stretching exercise for the leg.

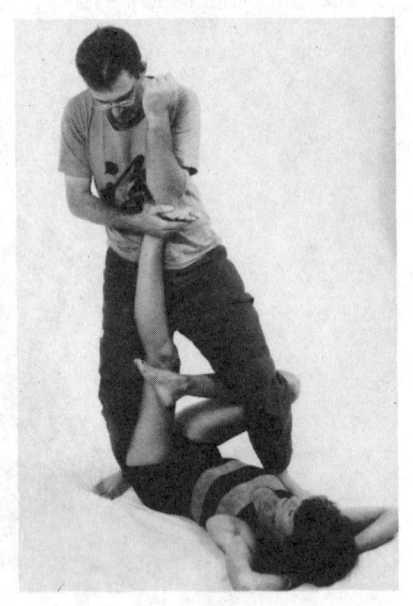

*Illustration 54*

This exercise can be extremely painful, which is why I've christened it 'The Spanish Inquisition'. (Doesn't it look like something right out of a torture chamber?) But the pain is of a kind that I would call 'good pain'. Such good pain results from hitting pressure points and vanishes as soon as the pressure is relaxed; good pain is invariably followed by a pleasant feeling of relief. 'Bad pain', on the other hand, results from mistakes of the masseur (e.g., pressing on bones, glands, etc.) and persists long after the pressure is lifted; bad pain has no positive effect on the body. Do your massage with mindfulness and concentration to avoid all such unnecessary pain—but you should definitely expect your patient to tolerate, even enjoy, a certain amount of 'good pain'.

Repeat the two exercises depicted in Illustration 53 and 54 with the other leg.

*A Whole-body Massage*

HEAD TO KNEES POSITION

Place the patient's legs on your body and grasp his arms at the wrists (Illustration 55). Ask the patient to grasp tightly around your wrists. (This prevents unnecessary and unhealthy pulling of the joints.) Pull the upper part of the body towards the knees. With flexible people the head will touch the knees.

If the patient is bigger than you it may be difficult to do this exercise with his legs straight in front of your body. In that case, place only his thighs on your legs and let the lower legs slide back behind your hips.

The exercise is excellent for the spine, the back and the shoulders.

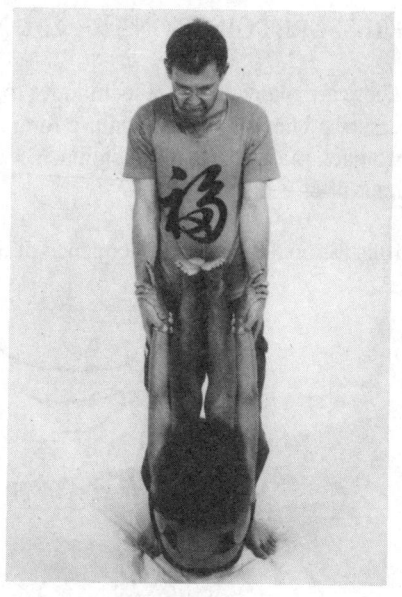

*Illustration 55*

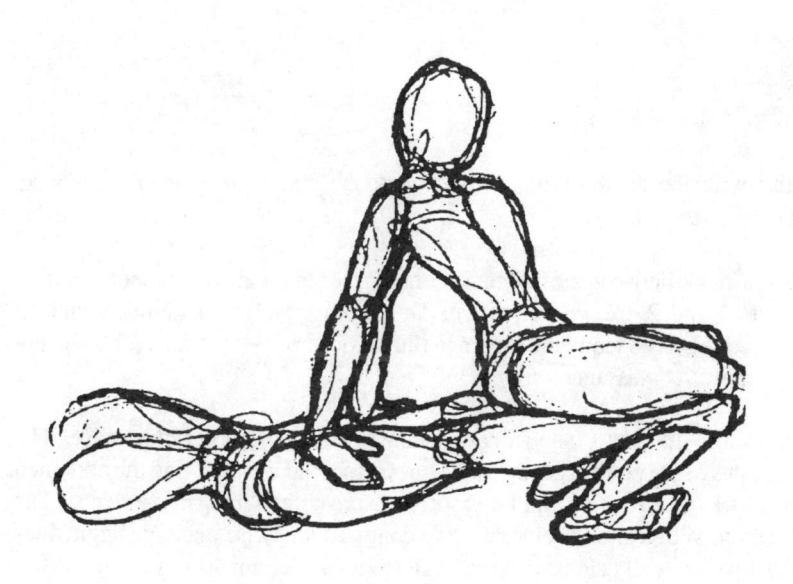

## 2.1.5 STOMACH MASSAGE

PRESSURE POINTS ON THE ABDOMEN

There are many different techniques to massage the abdomen. The technique described here is one I often use for a general, relaxing massage. Don't give stomach massage on a full stomach. Wait for 2-3 hours after a full meal or 1 hour after a snack.

Illustration 56 shows the sequence of the massage.

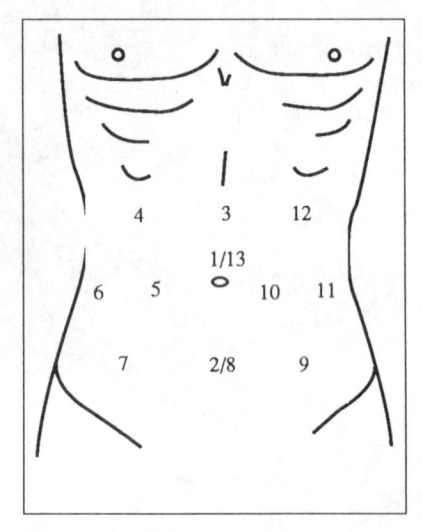

*Illustration 56*

Start with the navel (Point 1) and work the abdomen counter-clockwise, following the numbers.

The distance between the indicated points is the length of your patient's thumb. Points 1 and 2 are worked twice. They correspond with Points 8 and 13 respectively. The sequence shown in Illustration 56 is meant for a relaxing, not a therapeutic, massage.

**Caution:** In case of constipation don't massage counter-clockwise. The locations of the points stay the same but you should work around the abdomen in a clockwise direction, applying soft pressure with rubbing movements. (The direction of digestion is clockwise so counter-clockwise massage aggravates constipation while clockwise massage stimulates elimination.)

## A Whole-body Massage

*Illustration 57*

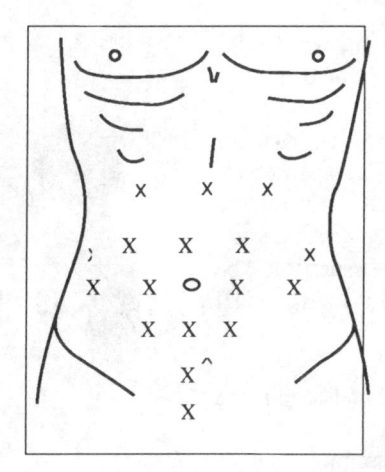

Illustration 57 is identical with the sequence in Illustration 56 except for two additional points below point 2/8. These new Points are therapy points for hernia, irregular or painful menstruation, excessive menstrual bleeding, etc.

## PALMING THE STOMACH

Carefully observe your patient's reactions. Push as far as you can get or until you notice even the slightest blinking in your partner's eyes.

The abdomen is one of the three main problem areas of many people, the other two being the lower back and the shoulders. Due to tension these areas are often extremely sensitive. Trust your intuition to enable you to give a soothing and calming massage.

Start by gently caressing the abdomen. Then do palming following the sequence given in Illustration 56. Use either hand-on-hand (as shown in Illustration 58) or only one hand for the palming. (One hand works better for very sensitive people.) Men may

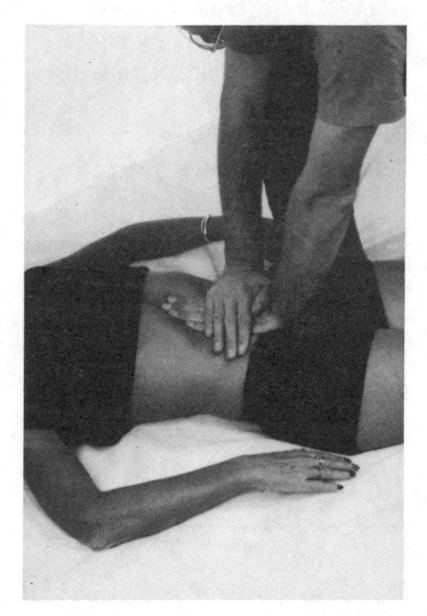

*Illustration 58*

55

have their legs straight, while with women the legs should be bent as in Illustration 59 to avoid unnecessary pressure on the ovaries. Always maintain the pressure for some seconds (up to 10 seconds) and then release slowly. No jerky movements! Pressure and the release of pressure must be done slowly and with full concentration.

Don't give a stomach massage if the patient is suffering from heavy abdominal pain. Massaging the lines on the back (they will be introduced later see Illustration 81) is much more helpful in such cases. Abdominal massage stimulates and relaxes internal organs and intestines for example:

*Illustration 59*

Point 1/13: Navel and intestines
Points 2/8, 7, 9 and 10: Intestines
Point 3: Stomach and solar-plexus
Point 4: Liver
Points 6 and 11: Kidneys
Point 12: Spleen and stomach.

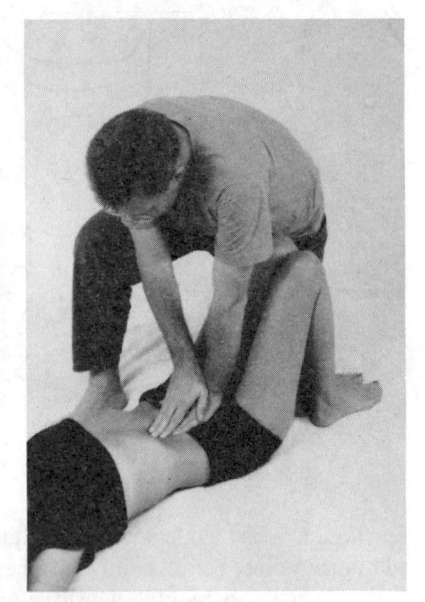

FINGER PRESSURE

In a second go-around apply pressure with your fingers as in Illustration 59. Take care that you don't work with your fingertips (and definitely not with your fingernails) but with the whole front part of your fingers. Follow the same sequence as in the palming but in this round always push towards the navel as you press.

## A Whole-body Massage

### THUMBING

Finish the abdominal massage with thumbing on the Point combinations of 4 and 12, 5 and 10, and 7 and 9. (See Illustration 60 and Illustration 56.) At the end do some gentle caressing movements all around the abdomen.

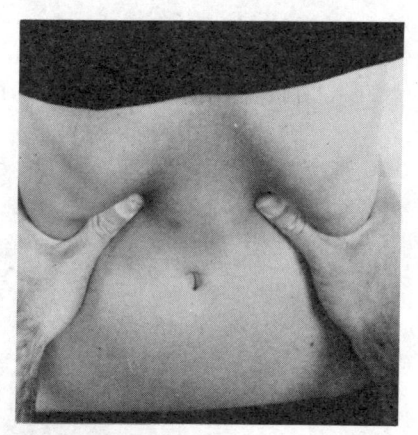

*Illustration 60*

---

### MASSAGE AND BREATHING

There is one aspect which is important throughout the whole massage but particularly important while massaging the abdomen. Your massage will be more profoundly satisfying and much more relaxing if you and your patient consciously observe some basic breathing rules.

During the abdominal massage whenever you press down your patient should exhale, thus releasing muscular tension and making it much easier for you to press.

You, on the other hand, should simultaneously inhale. When you release the pressure, your patient should inhale while you exhale. Whenever you hold a position, the patient should hold his breath. This breathing pattern (the masseur presses, pushes or pulls while inhaling and releases pressure while exhaling; the patient receives pressure while exhaling and when pressure is released, the patient is inhaling) is equally good for all stretching exercises as well. Synchronized breathing helps to relieve tension and supports the energy flow.

Other breathing patterns are also possible. One rhythm used very often is to combine the breathing of patient and masseur. While the masseur is pressing or pulling, both are breathing out. Both then breathe in again, when pressure or pull is released. Experiment and find out which pattern suits you most.

To coordinate the breathing of masseur and patient in this way increases the sensitivity on both sides. Ideally, perfect harmony will be created between masseur and patient. Give it a try and you will find a remarkable difference compared with a massage where coordination of breathing is not observed.

## 2.1.6 CHEST AND ARMS

### RELAXATION OF CHEST AND SHOULDERS

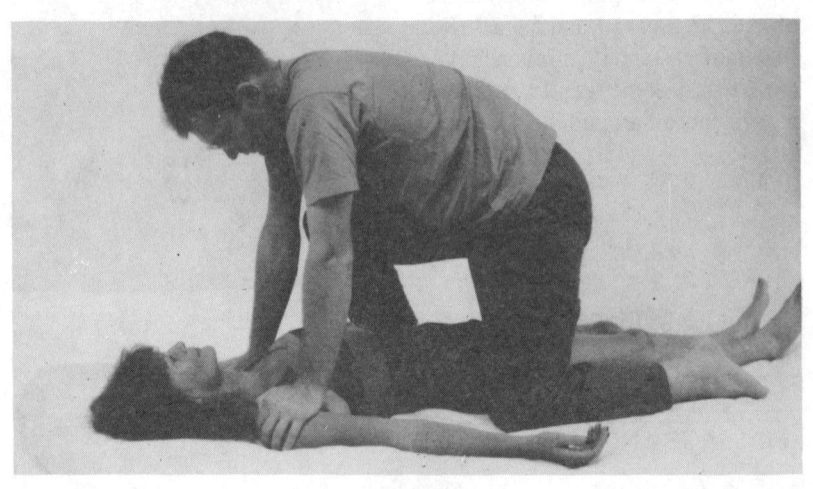

*Illustration 61*

Do some palming up and down the chest. Use your body weight for pressure. Press the soft depression at the shoulders (Illustration 61). When massaging women don't press on the breasts (which are very sensitive tissue) but only up and down the rib cage.

Work up and down the chest with the middle finger of one hand on the sternum, index finger and ring finger between the ribs. This stimulates *Sen Sumana*, one of the main energy lines.

### STOPPING THE BLOOD FLOW IN THE ARM

Grasp around the whole inside of the upper arm with your palm and hand and apply pressure with your body weight (Illustration 62). Hold for 20-30 seconds. You are stopping the blood flow from the arm to the fingertips. Slowly release the pressure. The sudden flow of blood cleans the blood

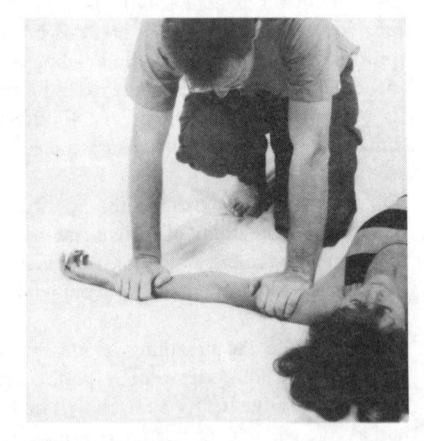

*Illustration 62*

## A Whole-body Massage

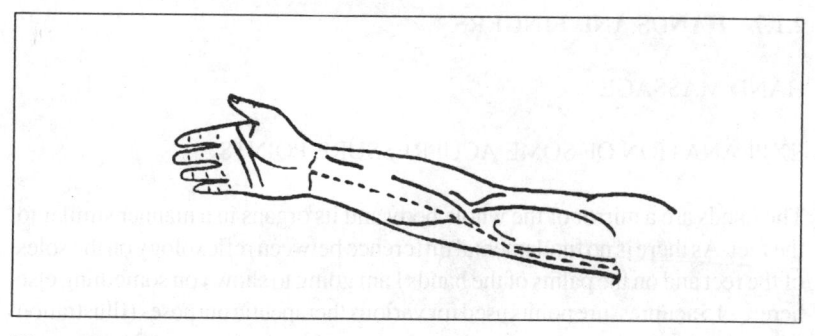

*Illustration 63*

vessels of dead cells and improves the blood circulation. Your hand on the lower arm holds without pressure.

**Caution:** Don't use in cases of hypertension or heart disease.

Do palming and thumbing along the middle line of the inside of the arm (depicted in Illustration 63). Take care, not to press on bone when you do thumbing. Work the line by pushing the biceps muscle upwards instead of pressing down with the thumbs. The line starts on the lower arm at the wrist and moves up to the elbow. On the upper arm the line runs below the front muscle (biceps) towards the armpit. (There is more than one line on the arm, but as the arm lines are difficult to locate, in this book I restrict myself to the main line.)

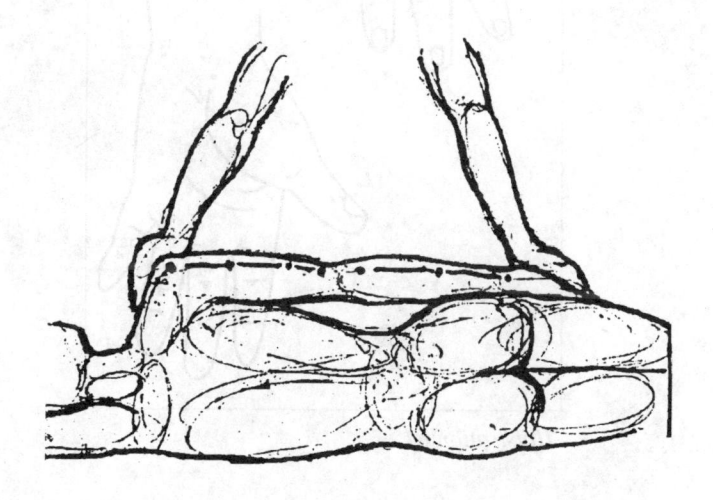

### 2.1.7 HANDS AND FINGERS

HAND MASSAGE

EXPLANATION OF SOME ACUPRESSURE POINTS

The hands are a mirror of the whole body and its organs in a manner similar to the feet. As there is no fundamental difference between reflexology on the soles of the feet and on the palms of the hands I am going to show you something else here:    15 acupressure points used for various therapeutic purposes (Illustration 64).

This is additional information on points not generally used in Thai massage. A detailed knowledge of these points is not necessary for a relaxing massage.

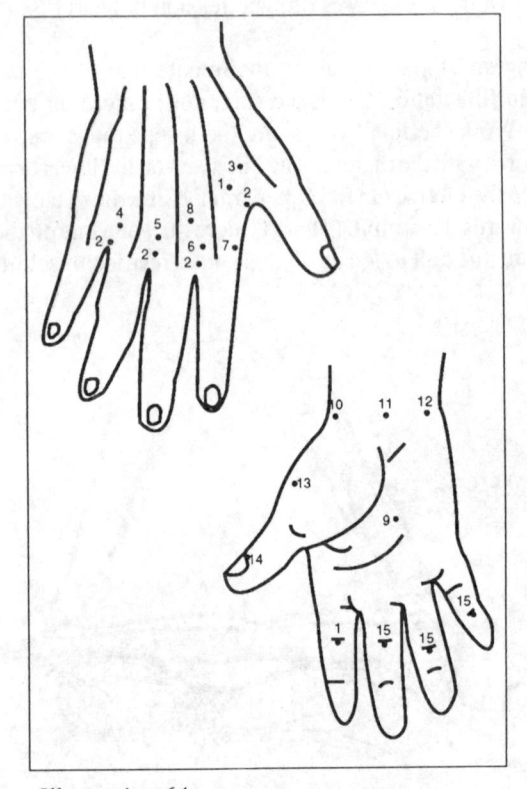

Illustration 64

*A Whole-body Massage*

## DORSUM OF THE HAND

**Point 1** is known as 'Hegu' in acupuncture and is one of the most important acupressure points. It is often called 'The Great Eliminator'. Pressing this point relieves all kinds of pain. Hegu is the harmless organic 'aspirin' which nature has provided for us. It is indicated for headache, abdominal pain, body ache and toothache. It also helps in cases of facial paralysis and common cold. To press Hegu is very painful, but it is 'good pain', bringing instant relief.

**Caution:** This point is prohibited for pregnant women. There is some danger that the 'Great Eliminator' could show its eliminating power here.

**Points 2 and 3**: For headache and toothache.

**Point 4**: For sciatic problems and pain in the hip.

**Point 5**: For sore throat and toothache.

**Point 6**: For stiffness in the neck.

**Point 7**: For pain in the shoulder and the shoulder joints.

**Point 8**: For stiffness in the neck, pain in the shoulder and arm, stomach pain, migraine, pain in the dorsum of the hand.

## PALM OF THE HAND

**Point 9**: For heat stroke and nausea.

**Point 10**: For asthma, chest pain, back and shoulder pain, diseases of the wrist.

**Point 11**: For diseases of the wrist, paralysis of the arm.

**Point 12**: For insomnia, dream-disturbed sleep, and angina pectoris.

**Point 13**: For cough, asthma, fever, sore throat, diseases of the tendon.

**Point 14**: For sore throat, fever, fainting, respiratory problems.

**Point 15**: For whooping cough and arthritis of the fingers.

There are innumerable exercises for massaging the hands and the fingers. Use your imagination. Wherever you press is fine—you can't do anything wrong. Play with the hands and fingers of your partner and trust your feelings. Let me just give you some suggestions:

*Illustration 65*

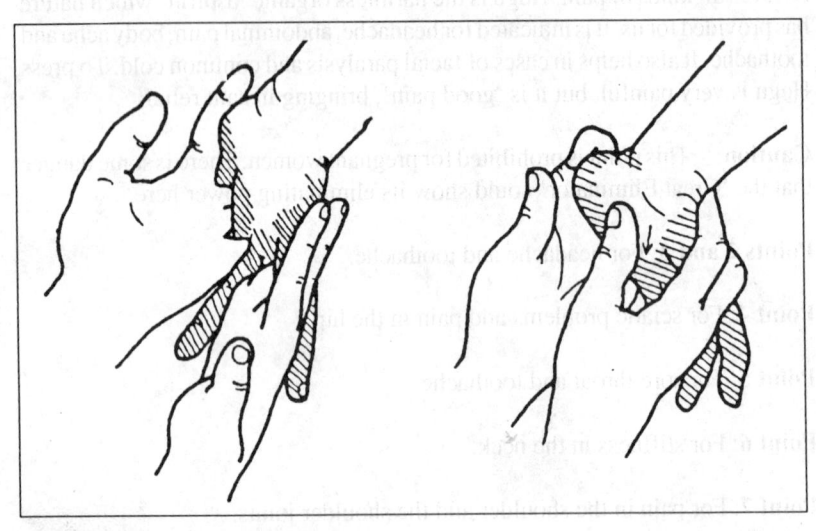

Illustration 65 shows how to interlace your patient's fingers with your fingers, sparing only his middle finger.

Do thumbing on the whole palm of the hand, at the same time push the hand downwards, applying pressure to the wrist.

Illustration 66 shows how to stretch the fingers.

It is also possible to form a fist with your patient's fingers and then grasp around and press.

Another very pleasant technique is to push the blood up the fingers to the fingertips. Simply let the thumb slide up the finger while giving good pressure. Do one finger after the other.

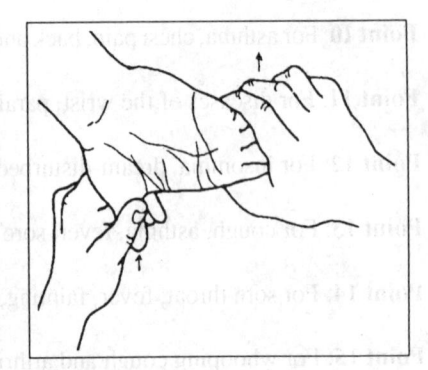

*Illustration 66*

## A Whole-body Massage

*Illustration 67*

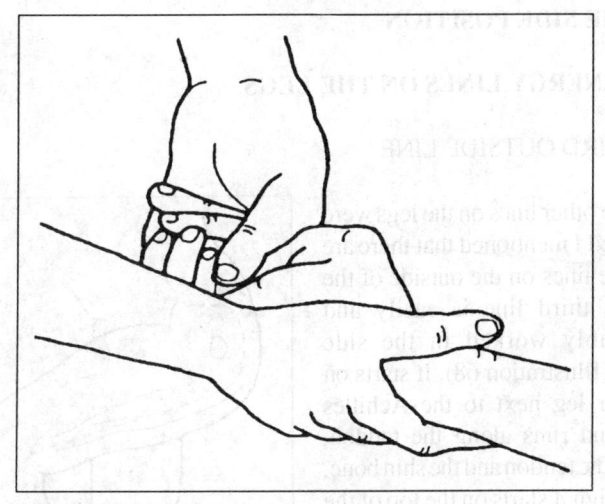

Illustration 67 shows how to stretch the straight fingers by grasping them with your hand.

After you've finished with one hand, repeat all the exercises with the other arm and hand, starting with Illustration 62.

## 2.2 THE SIDE POSITION

### 2.2.1 ENERGY LINES ON THE LEGS

THE THIRD OUTSIDE LINE

When the other lines on the legs were introduced I mentioned that there are also three lines on the outside of the leg. The third line is easily and comfortably worked in the side position (Illustration 68). It starts on the lower leg next to the Achilles tendon and runs along the tendon, between the tendon and the shin bone. On the thigh it starts on the top of the tendon at the side of the knee and runs right above the tendon.

The extension of the line across the buttock leads to the pelvis. In the pelvic area the line includes some very painful points which are used in massage therapy for cases of leg paralysis and for pain in the lower back.

If you have plenty of time, or if you are not doing a whole body massage, or if your patient needs an intensive workout on the energy lines (let's say for pain in the legs, fatigue, or disrupted energy flow), then it is also possible to do all the other energy lines on the legs in the side position. It's always good to do the lines—you can never do too much. (Use the techniques for palming and thumbing described earlier.)

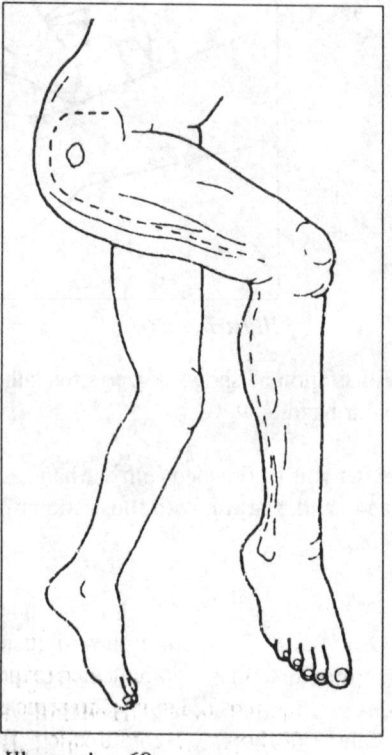

*Illustration 68*

Maintain the leg posture shown in Illustration 68 for the whole massage in the side position.

A Whole-body Massage

## 2.2.2 STRETCHING

STRETCHING OF ARM AND ARMPIT

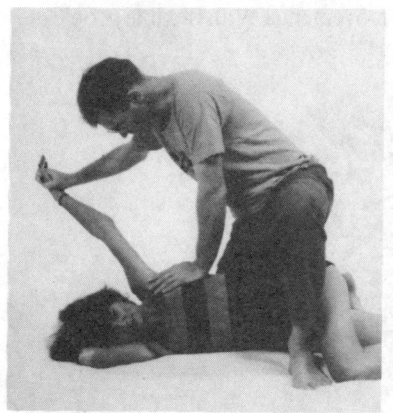

*Illustration 69*

*Illustration 70*

You are kneeling with one leg, stabilizing the back of the patient close to the shoulders. The other leg is bent in rectangular position. Interlace the patient's fingers with one hand, and with your other hand do palming up and down the arm, the armpit and the ribs (Illustration 69). Whenever you apply palm pressure, push the arm straight towards the patient's head. Don't press in the centre of the armpit but restrict yourself to working up and down the edge of it only.

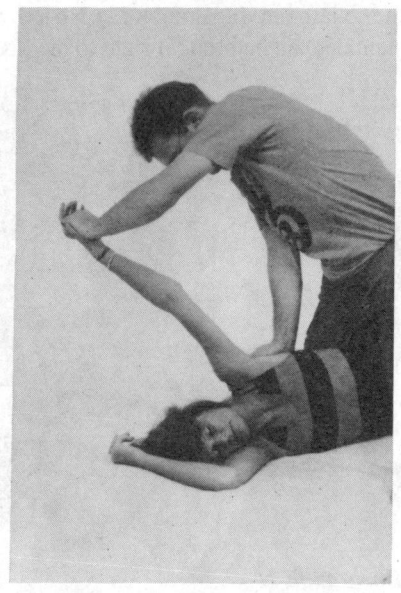

Change hands and work the other side (Illustration 70).

**Caution:** For some patients this exercise will be quite painful, and this pain can be difficult for the masseur to perceive.

## SPINAL TWIST

Fix the patient's bent leg with one hand. Slowly push the shoulder towards the floor with your other hand. Your palm must be placed in the depression below the collarbone (Illustration 71). No jerky movements! With flexible people the shoulder can be brought right to the floor.

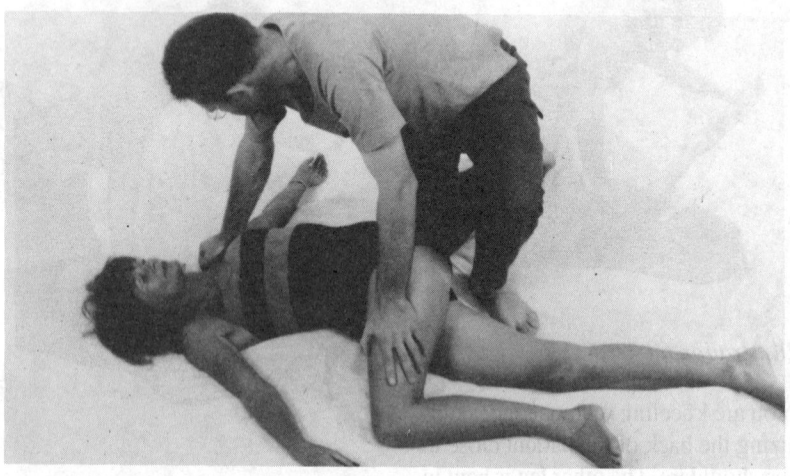

*Illustration 71*

We now come to a series of exercises (shown in Illustrations 72 to 75) which require a certain basic flexibility of the patient. These exercises are hard physical work for the masseur. Decide when and with whom you want to try these exercises.

Place your knee in the kidney area of the patient.

**Caution:** Don't put your knee on the ribs. If you feel bone you are doing it wrong.

The patient's hand and his lower arm are brought behind your back. Grasp around the knee with both hands, hand to hand. The lower leg is placed on your arm. Pull the leg slightly upwards and at the same time towards your body, which is bent back a bit (Illustration 72). Hold for a few seconds and release the pull.

If you like, you can place your knee further down at the buttock or the upper part of the thigh though this is not compulsory.

A Whole-body Massage

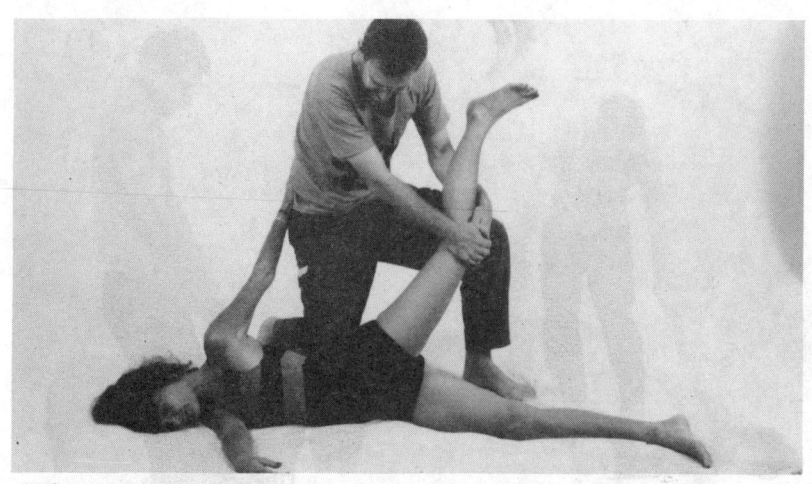

*Illustration 72*

Variation: Instead of standing, as in Illustration 72, you can kneel. This posture makes the exercise less effective, but it is also less strenuous for both you and your patient. Kneeling is ideal for working with stiff patients or very heavy people.

The stretches for the legs and the back depicted in Illustrations 73 and 74 are very similar. So the choice is up to you.

Grasp the arm of the patient at the wrist while the patient grasps and holds your wrist. Hold his foot and leg at the ankle. Your foot is fixing the kidney area (taking care not to touch bone). Lift the leg, pulling it up and slightly towards your body (Illustration 73). The pull is on the leg only, not on the arm which is merely held.

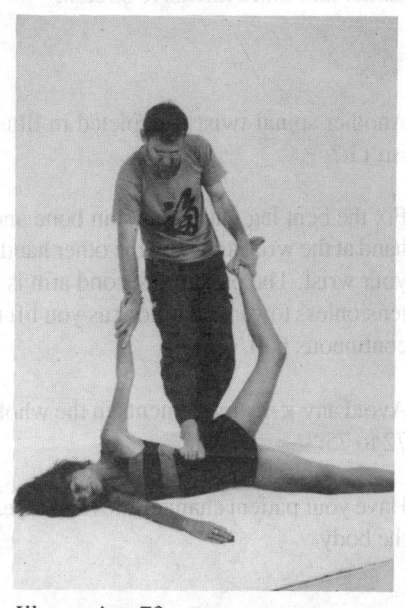

*Illustration 73*

67

*The Art of Traditional Thai Massage*

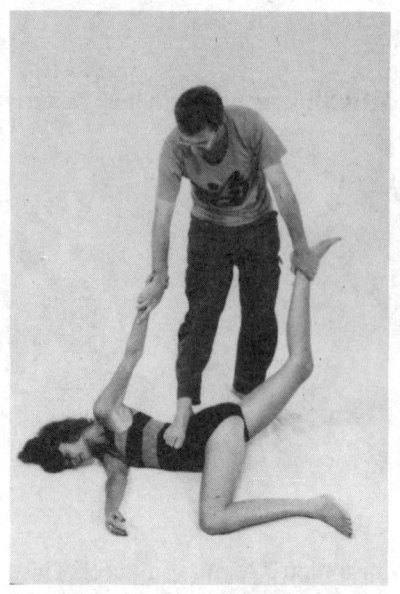

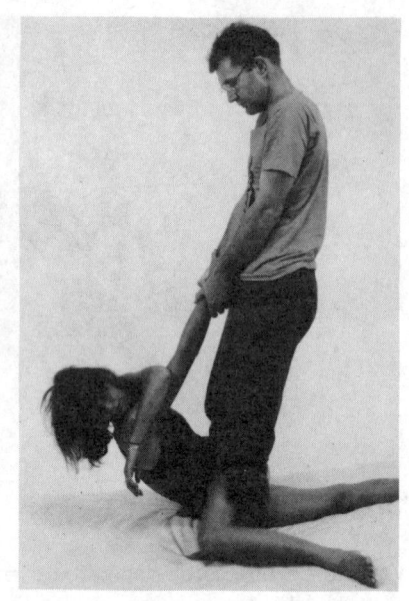

*Illustration 74*

*Illustration 75*

The variation in Illustration 74 is that you pull the other leg, which gives a harder and more intensive stretch.

Another spinal-twist is depicted in Illustration 75. What a beautiful posture, isn't it?

Fix the bent leg with your shin bone and grasp the arm on the floor with one hand at the wrist and with the other hand at the arm. Have your patient holding your wrist. The patient's second arm is placed on top of the other and moves tensionless towards the floor as you lift the upper part of the body with a slow continuous pull.

Avoid any jerky movements in the whole series of exercises from Illustration 72 to 75.

Have your patient change sides and repeat all the exercises on the other side of the body.

*A Whole-body Massage*

## 2.3 THE BACK PART OF THE BODY

### 2.3.1 FEET AND LEGS

THE LINES ON THE LEGS

Before you start with the exercises, you could work the lines on the legs in this position as well. The third inside line and the third outside line are very convenient to work. The first and the second inside lines are also possible, while the first and second outside line are difficult to reach. A workout on the lines in this position is not essential in a whole-body massage.

LOOSENING UP OF THE FEET AND FOOT JOINTS

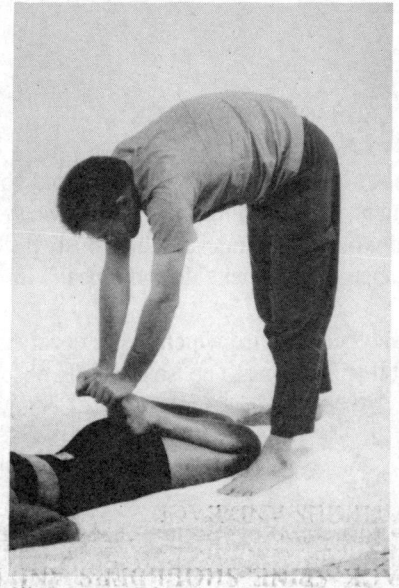

*Illustration 76*

Bend both the patient's legs, grasp around the toes, and then push towards the buttocks (Illustration 76). This is similar to the front-position exercise explained with Illustration 6; the exercises introduced with Illustration 7 and Illustration 8 and 9 can also be repeated here.

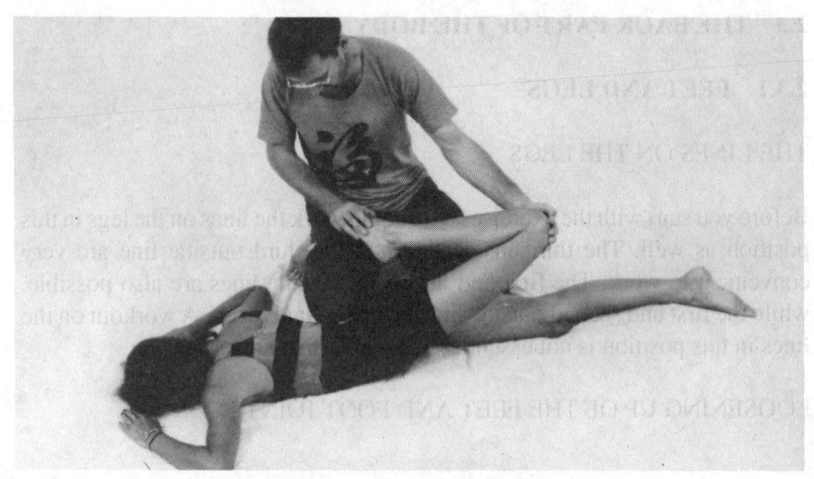

*Illustration 77*

## STRETCHING OF LEGS, HIP, AND BACK

Your knee is fixing the kidney area while with one hand you grasp around the bent knee of your patient. With the other hand push down the toes. Pull the bent leg slowly up towards your body while simultaneously pushing down the foot (Illustration 77). Change to the other side and repeat with the other leg.

**Caution:** This is another exercise which easily deceives the masseur. It is much more stressful than it seems to be, so carefully observe the reaction of your patient.

## THE 'LOCUST'

Illustration 78 shows a classical Yoga posture, the Shalabha Asana or 'Locust'.

Sit very lightly on the buttocks or the lower back of your patient, giving only enough pressure to fix his body. Grasp around the knee of one leg with both of your hands, fingers interlaced. Slowly lift the leg. As it is difficult to look into your patient's eyes in this position, ask him to tell you immediately when you reach the limit.

Repeat with the other leg.

Then with both legs together.

## A Whole-body Massage

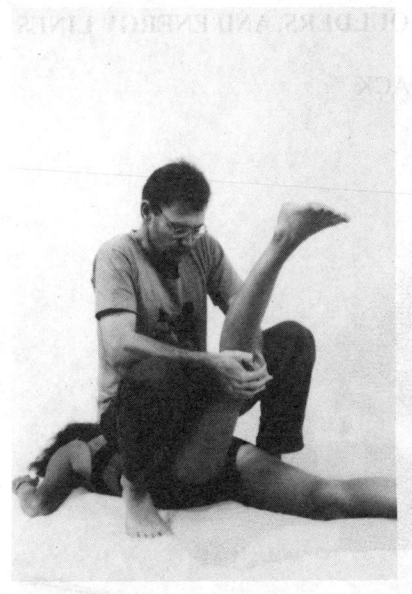

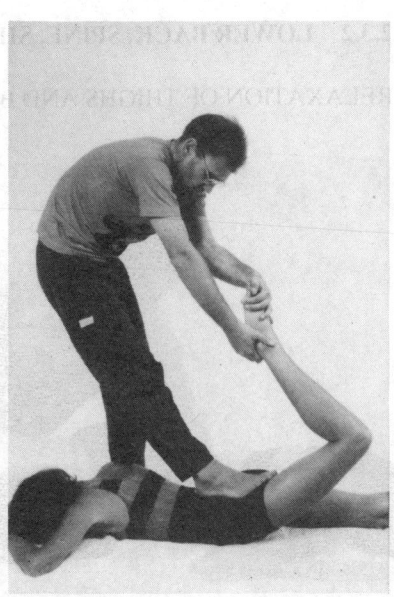

*Illustration 78*          *Illustration 79*

This exercise is extremely arduous physical work for the masseur. If you are massaging a person bigger and heavier than you, skip it if you feel it's too much.

The 'Locust' is an excellent therapy and prevention for hernia and strengthens abdominal and pelvic muscles.

There is another exercise similar to the 'Locust' (Illustration 79). Lift the bent leg of the patient, pulling upwards and towards your body, while fixing the buttock with your foot, and holding the patient's foot at the heel and at the toes. Your other leg is placed at the level of his armpit.

Repeat with the other leg.

## 2.3.2 LOWER BACK, SPINE, SHOULDERS, AND ENERGY LINES

RELAXATION OF THIGHS AND BACK

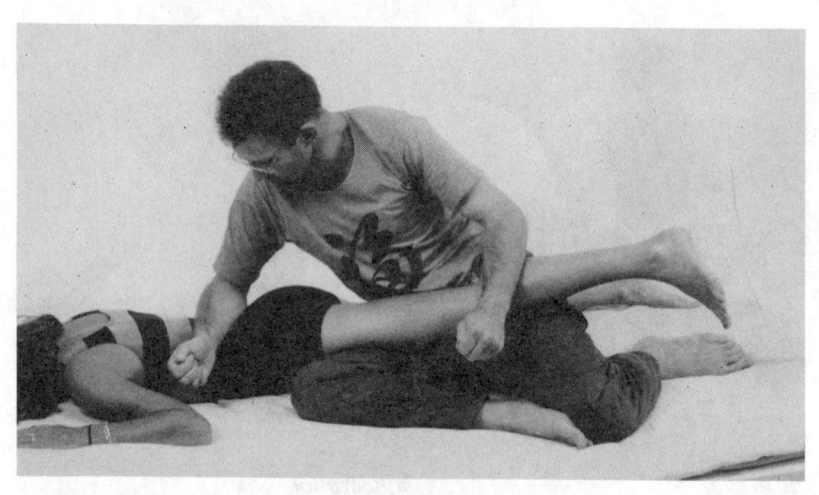

*Illustration 80*

Sit between your patient's legs. One of your legs is bent backwards, the other one is bent in front of your body. The patient's leg is placed on your thigh while your bent leg is near the patient's pelvic region. Roll your arm up and down the thigh, the buttock, and the back. Roll your other arm up and down the calf (Illustration 80).

Change to the other side and repeat.

*A Whole-body Massage*

## THE ENERGY LINES ON THE BACK

*Illustration 81*

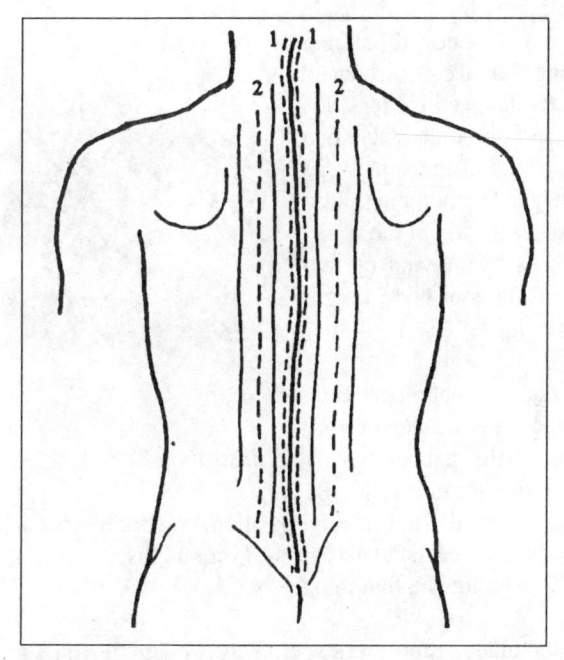

Illustration 81 shows the running of two of the main energy lines on the back.

**Line 1** runs on both sides next to the spine.

**Line 2** also runs on both sides of the spine but at a distance of one thumb length outward from line one (the thumb measure of your patient). You can feel the running of a muscle (muscular ridge) there.

The energy lines on the back are connected with more or less all the organs and body functions. These lines are especially effective for the treatment of stomach problems, diseases of the liver, the gall bladder, the spleen, the bladder and the kidneys as well as for pain and problems of the back and the shoulders. In all these cases an intensive workout on the back lines can bring noticeable relief.

It's always a good idea to do the back lines again and again. There's nothing you can do wrong, and your work will benefit your patient's whole body.

## WORKING THE ENERGY LINES

To work the energy lines on the back, use the same techniques of palming and thumbing that were introduced earlier with the lines on the legs. Do palming up and down the back, one hand on each side of the spine. Use your body weight. For thumbing, place one thumb on each side of the spine. Cover the lines by moving up and down while using your body weight to apply pressure.

You can work in a kneeling position, your body either to one side of your patient or with the patient's body between your thighs. Illustration 82 shows a truly 'classical' Thai massage position for working the back. Sit on the soles of your patient's feet. Put his hands on your thighs above the knees. Work the lines with palming and thumbing.

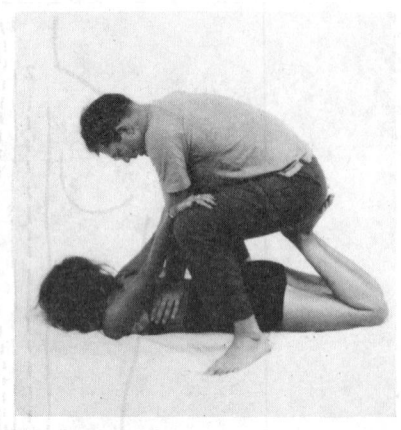

*Illustration 82*

Also use your imagination and experiment a bit until you find a posture comfortable for you.

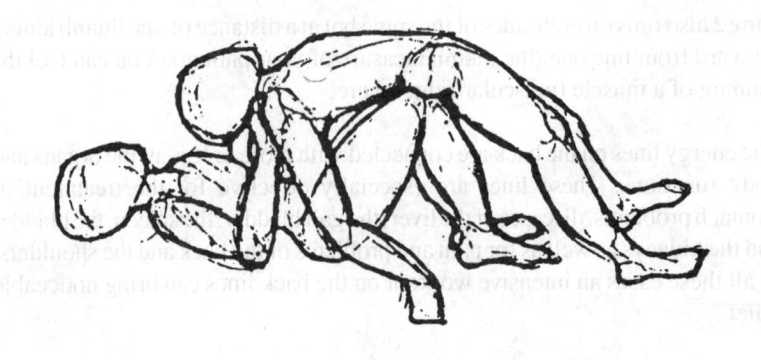

*A Whole-body Massage*

## 2.3.3 'COBRA' STRETCHES

The 'Cobra' posture comes from the Yoga tradition and in Sanskrit it is called Bhujanga Asana. In Thai massage as well as in Yoga there is a multitude of variations, of which three will be introduced here.

The 'Cobras' are excellent for treating tension in the lower back, the neck, and the shoulder area. They are also a powerful spinal exercise, benefiting the whole spine.

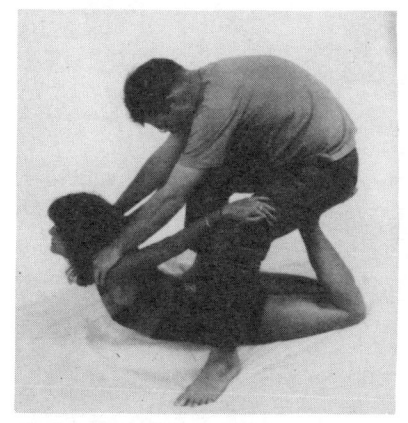

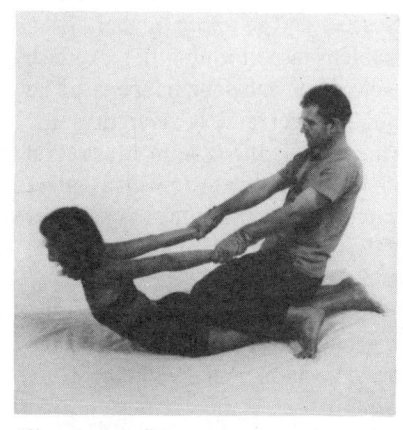

*Illustration 83*                    *Illustration 84*

For the exercise in Illustration 83 use the same starting position as in Illustration 82. Grasp around the shoulders and slowly lift up the patient. (No jerky movements please!) Hold the position for some seconds. Bring the upper part of the body gently back to the floor. This Cobra is good for stiff and heavy people.

Kneel on the thighs of your patient. Grasp the arms at the wrists and have the patient grasp your arms. Lift up slowly (Illustration 84). This is the "standard" 'Cobra' for use with most people. In your massage practice, you will most probably often opt for this variation. You may skip the others then.

You can vary the effect on the spine by fixing with your knees higher or lower on your patient's thighs. Take care to keep some distance from the knees.

Illustration 85 shows the same exercise but you are standing on the thighs, which again alters the effect on back and spine. First, grasp the patient's arms before standing on the thighs. This will help you to keep balance. Skip the exercise if your position is not firm and stable.

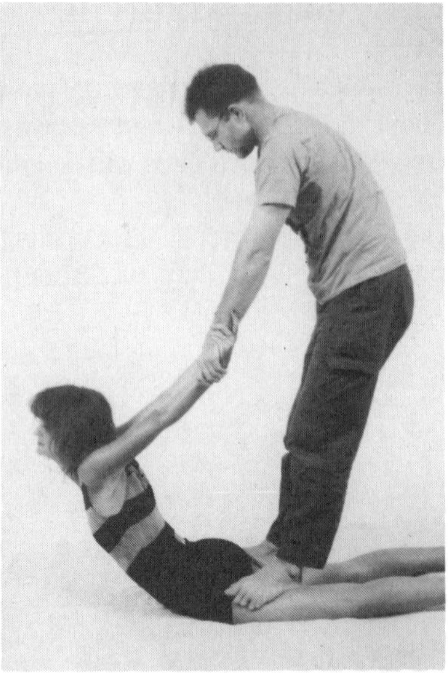

The thighs can stand quite a lot of pressure and so normally there is no problem in performing this exercise even if the masseur happens to be much bigger and heavier than the patient, as is the case in Illustration 85. But it is easier to do with a patient heavier than you are, as the patient's body weight stabilizing the position then.

*Illustration 85*

We conclude the back exercises in the prone position with a variation of the 'Locust'.

Hold both legs at the foot joints. Place your foot on the coccyx (Illustration 86) but apply only enough pressure to fix the coccyx. Lift the legs. Hold for some seconds and then release. Now place your foot across the spine at the lower back, then below the shoulder blades, repeating the lift-up in each position.

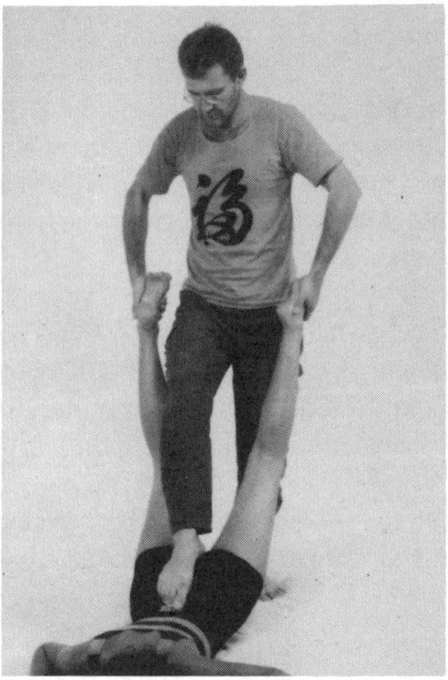

**Caution:** Don't step on the spine with the heel or the ball of the foot; The vertebrae must be bridged by the arch in the centre of the foot. Avoid all strong pressure on the spine. Take care that all the pressure applied in this exercise comes from your lifting of the patient's legs—not from your foot and your body weight.

*Illustration 86*

*A Whole-body Massage*

## 2.4  THE SITTING POSITION

### 2.4.1  SIT-UPS

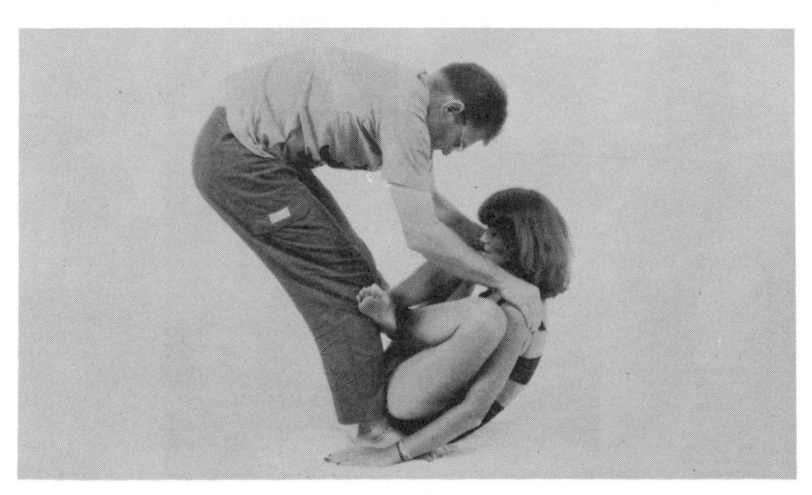

*Illustration 87*

Ask your patient to turn over so that he is lying on his back.

Cross his legs 'Indian style' (Sukha Asana or the 'Tailor's Seat') and place them on your shin bone below your knees (Illustration 87). Flexible people may be lifted up at the shoulders, which is strenuous work for the masseur but a good counter-exercise to the 'Cobra'.

Skip this exercise with stiff people or with patients too heavy for you to handle.

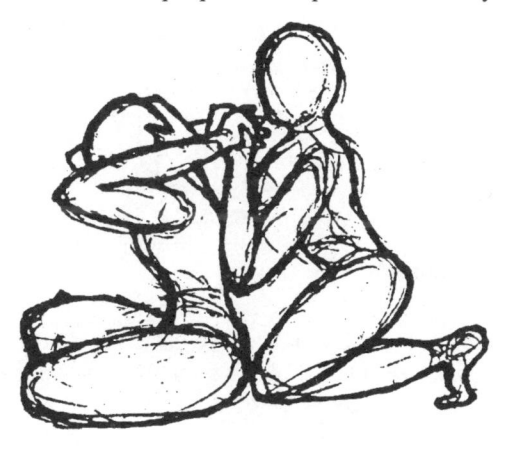

77

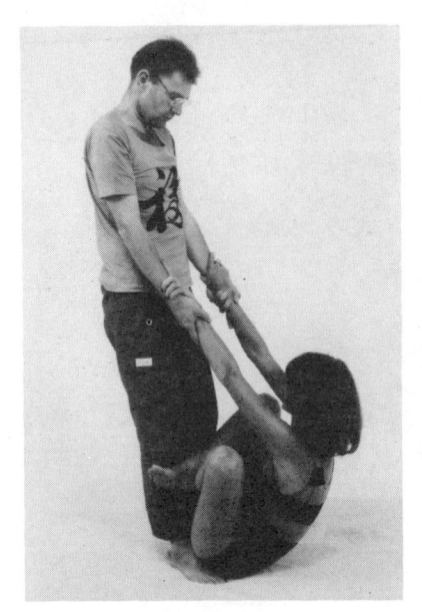

# The Art of Traditional Thai Massage

*Illustration 88* 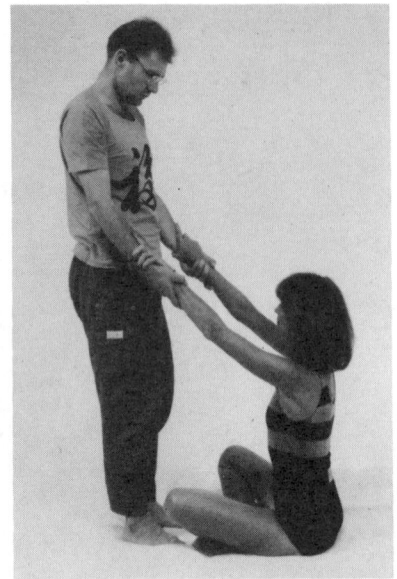  *Illustration 89*

Having completed the exercise depicted in Illustration 87 (or perhaps instead of it), grasp the patient's arms at the wrists and pull him up on his arms (Illustration 88). Do the pull-up two or three times and then walk back and bring the patient to a sitting position (Illustration 89).

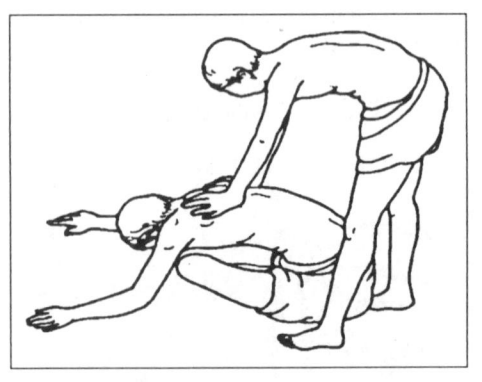

Illustration 90

Push the patient's torso down with your body weight as depicted in Illustration 90. Do palming on the back lines. This is a good counter-exercise to the 'Cobras', creating a perfect balance.

A *Whole-body Massage*

## 2.4.2 ARMS, SHOULDERS, AND SHOULDER BLADES

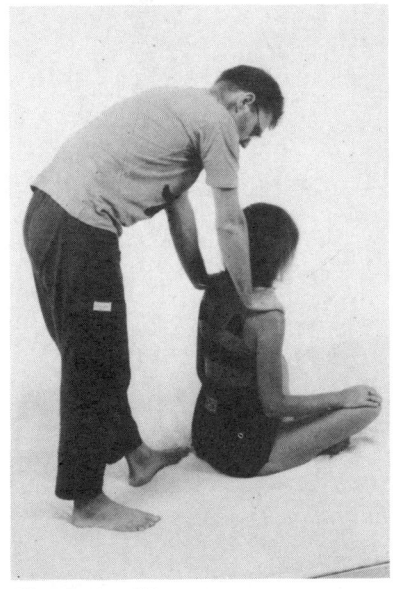

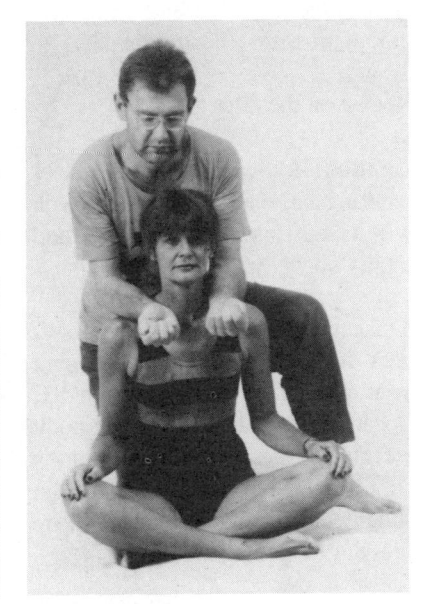

*Illustration 91*                *Illustration 92*

All kinds of problems and worries tense up the shoulders. So the shoulder massage can do a lot of good.

Sit the patient straight up and do palming on the shoulders (Illustration 91).

**Caution:** Don't press on bones. With many people the shoulders are extremely tense and very sensitive. Often even the slightest pressure causes terrible pain.

Roll your lower arms on the shoulders as shown in Illustration 92. (Take care again not to work on bones.)

Push the head to the side with one hand. Locate with your elbow the soft area on the shoulders and then apply elbow-pressure (Illustration 93).

Repeat on the other side.

**Caution**: If you make the mistake of working the bones in this exercise you will create lasting, unhealthy, and totally unnecessary pain.

You can also do thumbing on the soft area of the shoulders. Stand behind your patient as in Illustration 91. Locate the soft area and, using body weight, press with both thumbs simultaneously on both sides of the shoulders. Cover the whole area by pressing several points.

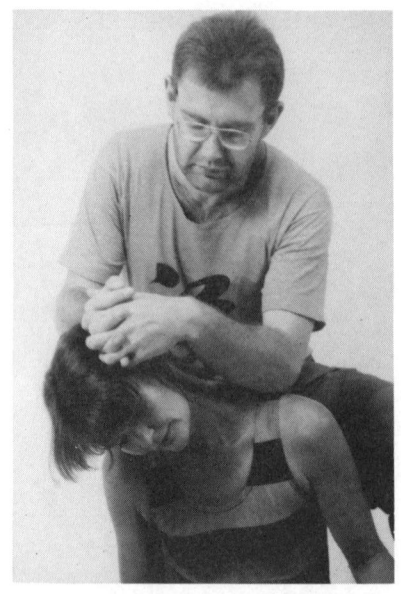

*Illustration 93*

**Caution**: With many people this area is very painful. Since it is 'good pain' loosening up tension you can expect your patient to bear a certain amount of pain—but don't overdo it.

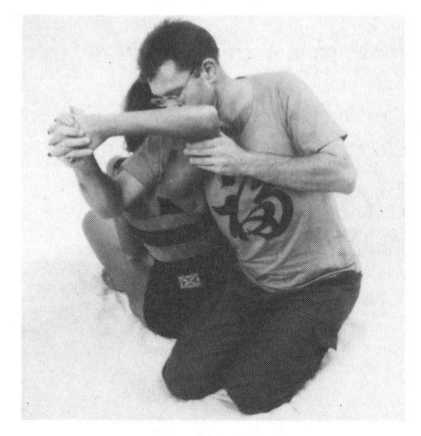

Illustration 94 shows an exercise for working the arm line. Kneel to the side of the patient, facing him. Interlace his fingers with the fingers of one of your hands. Place the upper arm across the shoulder and stretch. With your other hand apply thumb pressure up and down the line on the upper arm (see Illustration 63), the edge of the armpit (not the centre!) and the ribs. In the upper arm you can feel a nerve stretched like a guitar string. If you pluck at the nerve the patient will feel an 'electric shock' up to the fingertips. This is good treatment for motion problems of the arm but don't play around with it too much (since it produces quite an unpleasant feeling.) So plucking it once is enough.

*Illustration 94*

## A Whole-body Massage

The problem in this exercise is the position of the masseur. You should not push the patient backwards or to the side but keep him straight and erect. Kneel as near as possible to the patient with the upper part of your upper arm covering the shoulder and stabilising the patient's straight seat. Place your knees as far as you can behind the patient.

If you find this exercise too difficult to handle I have an alternative for you. Illustration 95 shows a simple variation which is not so elegant but much easier to do.

Bend the patient's arm and put his hand on his shoulder. With one hand pull back on his elbow with the other hand work the arm line.

*Illustration 95*

### LOOSENING-UP OF THE SHOULDERS

Kneel behind the patient. Grasp the wrist of the bent arm with one hand, and with the other hand hold the fingers. The elbow of your arm which is holding the wrist works up and down the back between spine and shoulder blade as your hand pulls back the arm of the patient. Your other hand doesn't have to pull but only supports the movement (Illustration 96).

**Caution:** Absolutely no pressure should be applied on the spine and shoulder blades. You can inflict lasting, unnecessary pain.

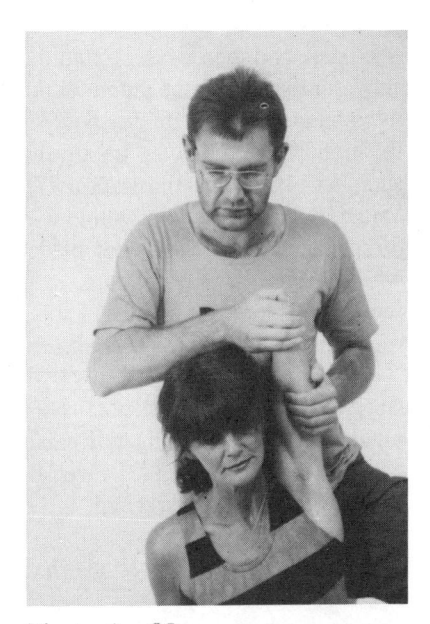

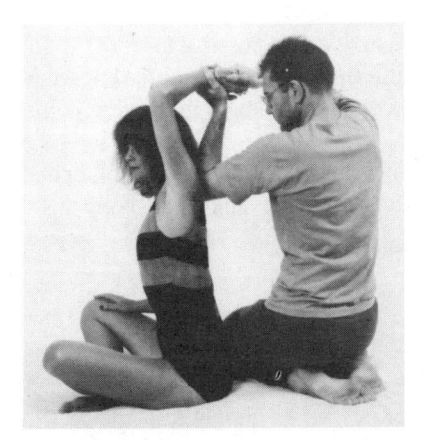

*Illustration 96*

## LOOSENING-UP OF THE SHOULDER BLADES

Kneel behind the patient. The patient's arm is bent towards the back, and the dorsum of the hand placed on the back. Fix the palm of the hand with your knee, grasp the shoulder with one hand, and then work around the shoulder blade with the thumb of the other hand. Pull back on the shoulder to support the opening up of the shoulder blade area (Illustration 97). With flexible people your thumb will disappear under the shoulder blade, while in tense people this area will seem to be more like a piece of solid rock where nothing moves at all.

But even in extreme cases of tension, regular massage will bring noticeable change after only a couple of weeks. Your partner will be surprised.

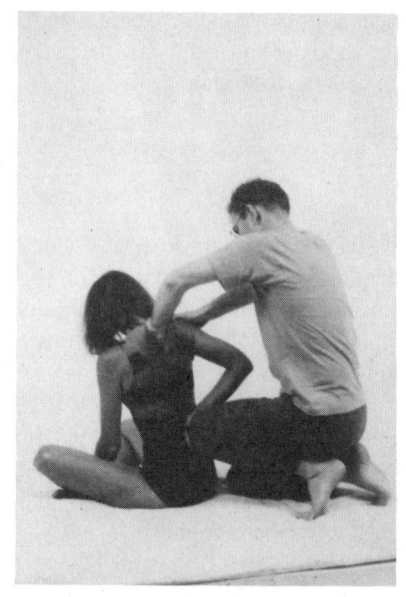

*Illustration 97*

After this exercise you may shake the arm to relax it. Hold the arm at the fingers.

Now repeat the exercises (starting with Illustration 94) on the other side of the body.

Note: It is also possible to work the lines on the back (see Illustration 81) in the sitting position. But since the line workout is easier in the prone position, I don't recommend doing it in the sitting position as part of a whole-body massage.

The sitting position is excellent for massaging pregnant women and, of course, when you give only a part-body massage.

*A Whole-body Massage*

### 2.4.3 HEAD AND NECK

LOOSENING-UP THE NECK VERTEBRAE

Place the patient's head between your lower arms, your hands folded 'prayer style'. (In Sanskrit this is called Namaskar Mudra.) Pull the head back gently and slowly as far as possible (Illustration 98). No jerky movements please.

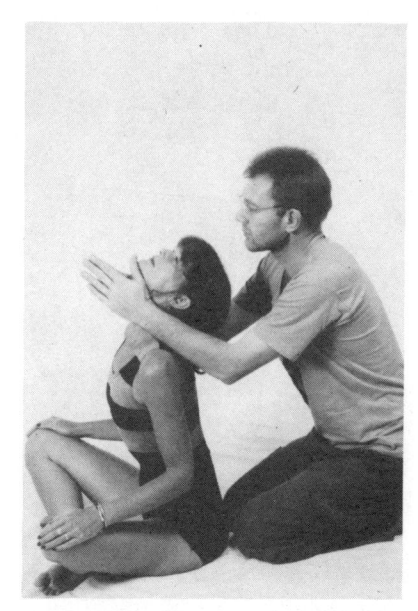

*Illustration 98*

Turn the head slowly to the side and pull back. (Illustration 99).

Repeat on the other side.

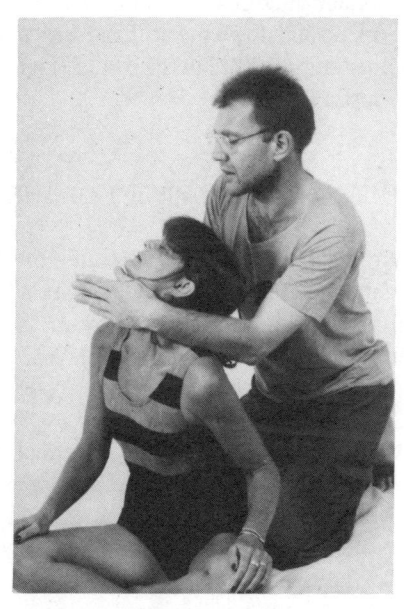

*Illustration 99*

## RELAXING THE NECK

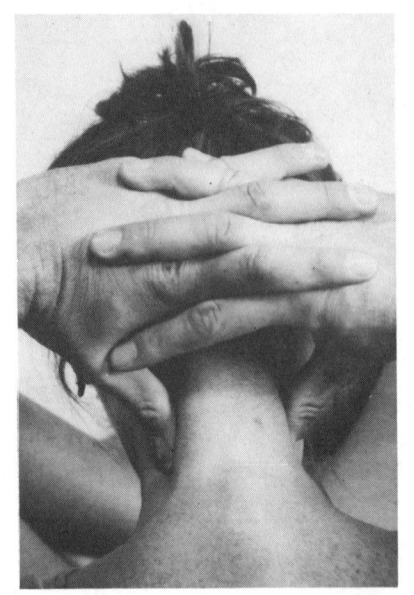

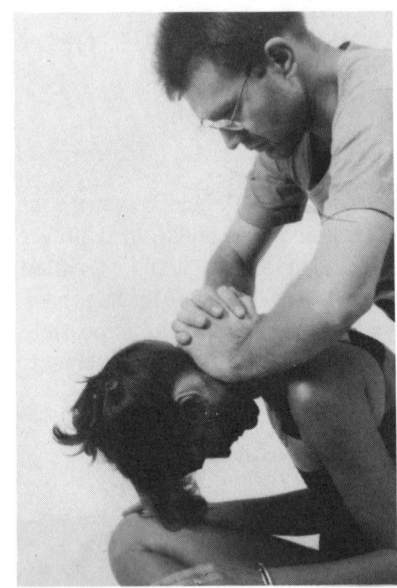

*Illustration 100*            *Illustration 101*

Interlace your fingers (using the same hand position as in Illustration 29) and work up and down the neck muscles (trapezius muscles) with thumb pressure (Illustration 100). Interlace your fingers and do palming on the neck muscles (Illustration 101).

## THE POSTERIOR ASPECT OF THE HEAD AND NECK

Work with thumb pressure (preferably thumb on thumb) along the middle line of the head as illustrated in Illustration 102. Start with **Point 1** in the depression directly below the base of the skull. (This is a therapy point for headache, stiff neck, and swelling of the throat). Working this line relaxes the head and brings relief from headache. The line stops right at the beginning of the forehead.

**Point 2** is one of the most important of the energy centres known in Yoga philosophy, the Seventh Chakra or Sahasara Chakra. This Chakra is our window to cosmic consciousness and it can be stimulated by massage. To locate the point, fold one ear and follow the tip of the fold up to the middle of the skull. There you will find a small depression, more or less obvious in different people.

*A Whole-body Massage*

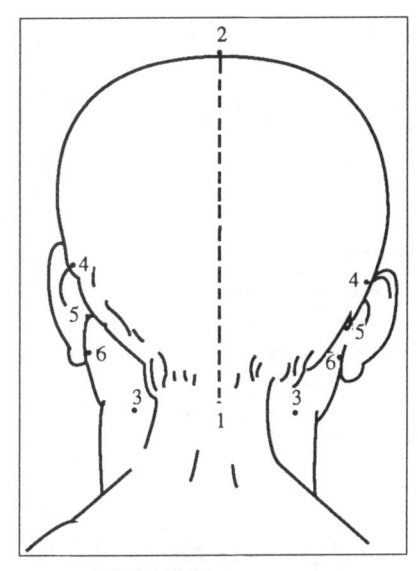

*Illustration 102*

**Points 3** are depressions slightly below the base of the skull. They are very sensitive to pressure and therefore easily located. These points are very effective for headache, but you may skip them in a general massage as they are very painful. Work them simultaneously with thumb pressure.

**Points 4, 5, and 6** lie at depressions directly behind the ears: Point 4 at the upper edge of the ears, Point 5 in the middle, Point 6 at the lower edge. These points are good for ear pain and ear diseases. You may also do them at the end of the massage as part of the face massage. Work with thumb pressure; I suggest rubbing, rotating movements of the thumbs.

**Caution:** Only soft pressure is allowed on Point 6. The artery to the brain runs below it and continuous strong pressure is dangerous! Don't work the middle line of the head and the Seventh Chakra on children less than 7 years of age!

In addition to the points mentioned here, also work with thumb pressure along the base of the skull. A good technique for that is to hold the patient's forehead with one hand while working with the thumb of the other hand from the centre of the base of the skull outwards and then back, pushing upwards with the thumb.

Then change hands and repeat on the other side.

85

*The Art of Traditional Thai Massage*

'SHAMPOOING'

Cover the whole scalp with jerky movements of your fingers (Illustration 103). This relaxes the scalp and strengthens the hair.

'PULLING HAIR'

An excellent exercise to strengthen the roots of the hair and to prevent baldness is 'pulling hair'. There are people who outrightly hate this exercise (suffering from a childhood trauma, maybe?). Skip it with those people. On the other hand you will find enthusiasts like myself who can't get enough of it.

**Caution:** Do this exercise on dry hair only. Wet hair (after taking a bath or heavy sweating) will easily break.

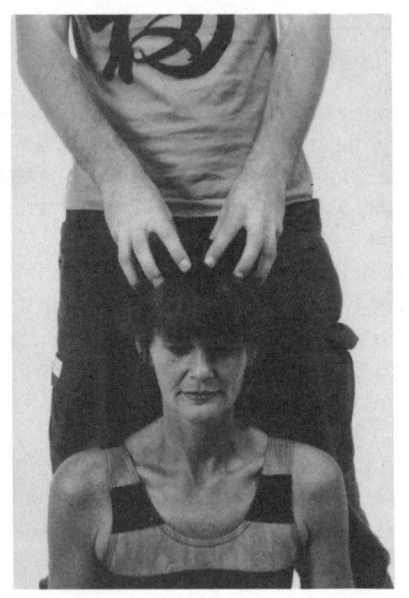

*Illustration 103*

*A Whole-body Massage*

## 2.4.4 STRETCHES

Stand behind the patient and stabilise his body. His interlaced hands are placed on the back of his head (not on the neck!). Grasp around the arms and pull the patient up by his upper arms. At the same time pull backwards at the elbow region with your lower arms (Illustration 104). You can repeat the exercise placing your hands at different spots along the patient's upper arms. Good for shoulders and arms.

**Caution:** This is another one of the exercises which might be overly rigorous and strenuous for the patient without the masseur realising it. Take it easy.

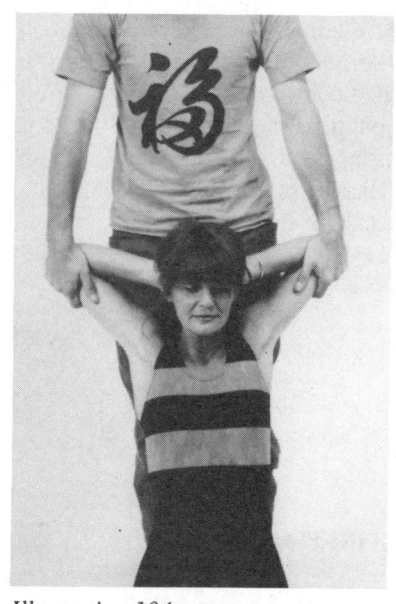

*Illustration 104*

The starting position for the patient in Illustration 105 is the same as in Illustration 104. Grasp through the space between your patient's upper and lower arms and hold the arms near the wrists as shown in Illustration 105. Work up and down his back next to the spine with your knees. Simultaneously pull back the patient on his arms whenever you press with your knees.

**Caution:** Don't hit the spine with your knees.

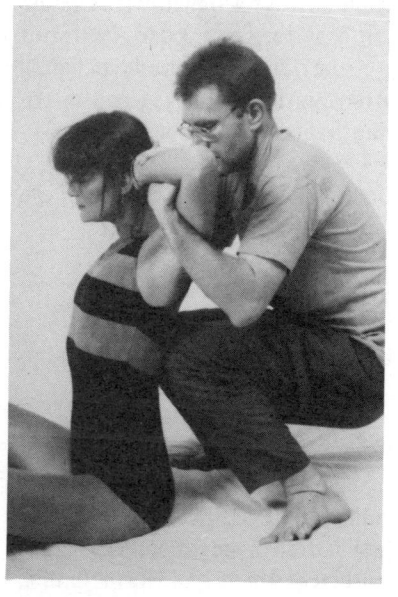

*Illustration 105*

The hand position of masseur and patient in Illustration 106 is the same as in the previous exercise (Illustration 105). One of the masseur's knees is on the floor, the other leg is bent. Push your patient's body towards the floor as far as it will comfortably go. With flexible people the head will easily touch the floor.

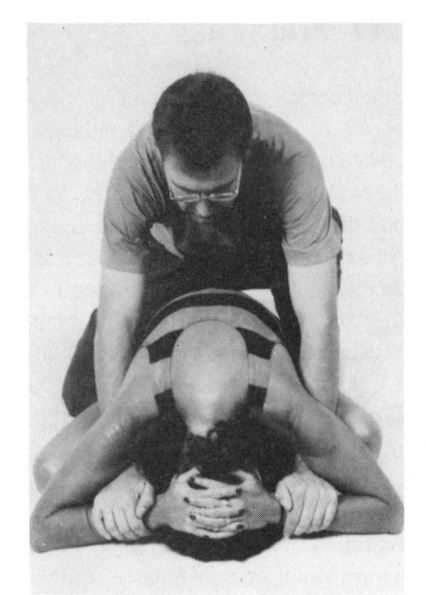

SPINAL TWIST

*Illustration 106*

After you have brought the patient back to an upright sitting position, it's again time for a spinal twist. Fix the thigh with your knee (without pressure), and then turn the patient's torso with a slow, firm move (Illustration 107). No jerks please!

You may hear some cracking of the spine.

Repeat to the other side.

**Caution:** Don't force this exercise on very stiff people.

With very flexible people, instead of fixing the thigh with your knee, stretch your leg out straight and place your foot in front of the patient's legs. This will give you more space for the turning movement.

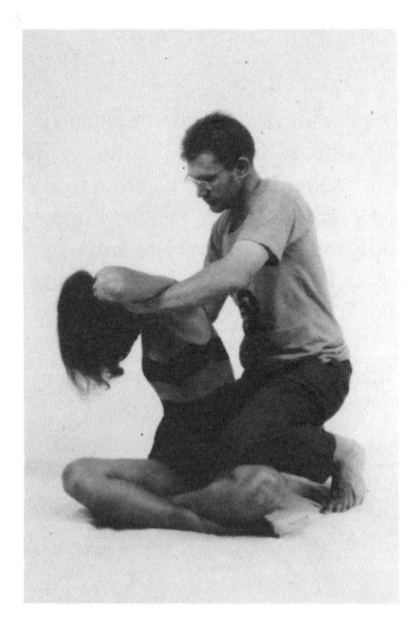

*Illustration 107*

A Whole-body Massage

WALKING ON THE BACK

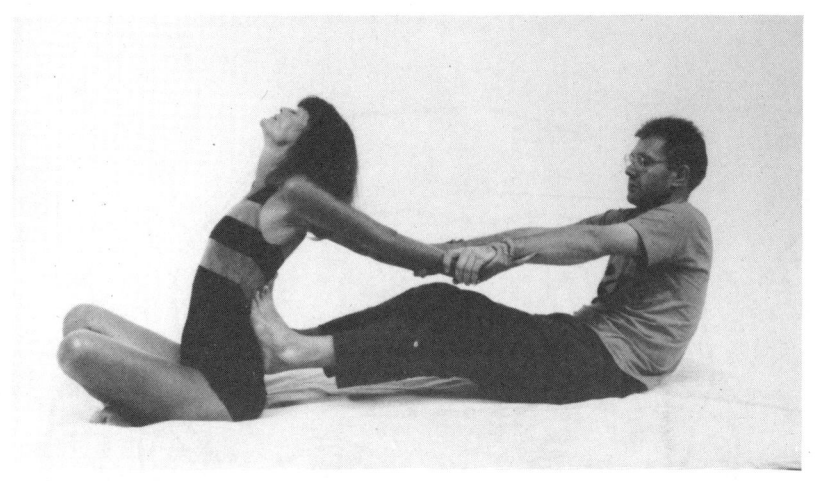

*Illustration 108*

Sit behind your patient and grasp his arms at the wrists, letting him hold your wrists (Illustration 108). Walk up and down his back next to the spine while simultaneously applying pressure with both legs. Whenever you push with your legs, use your body weight to pull the patient back on his arms.

**Caution:**   Don't walk on the spine but rather next to it.

Close the workout in the sitting position by repeating the exercise shown in Illustration 90, pushing forward the upper part of the body.

## 2.5 THE FACE

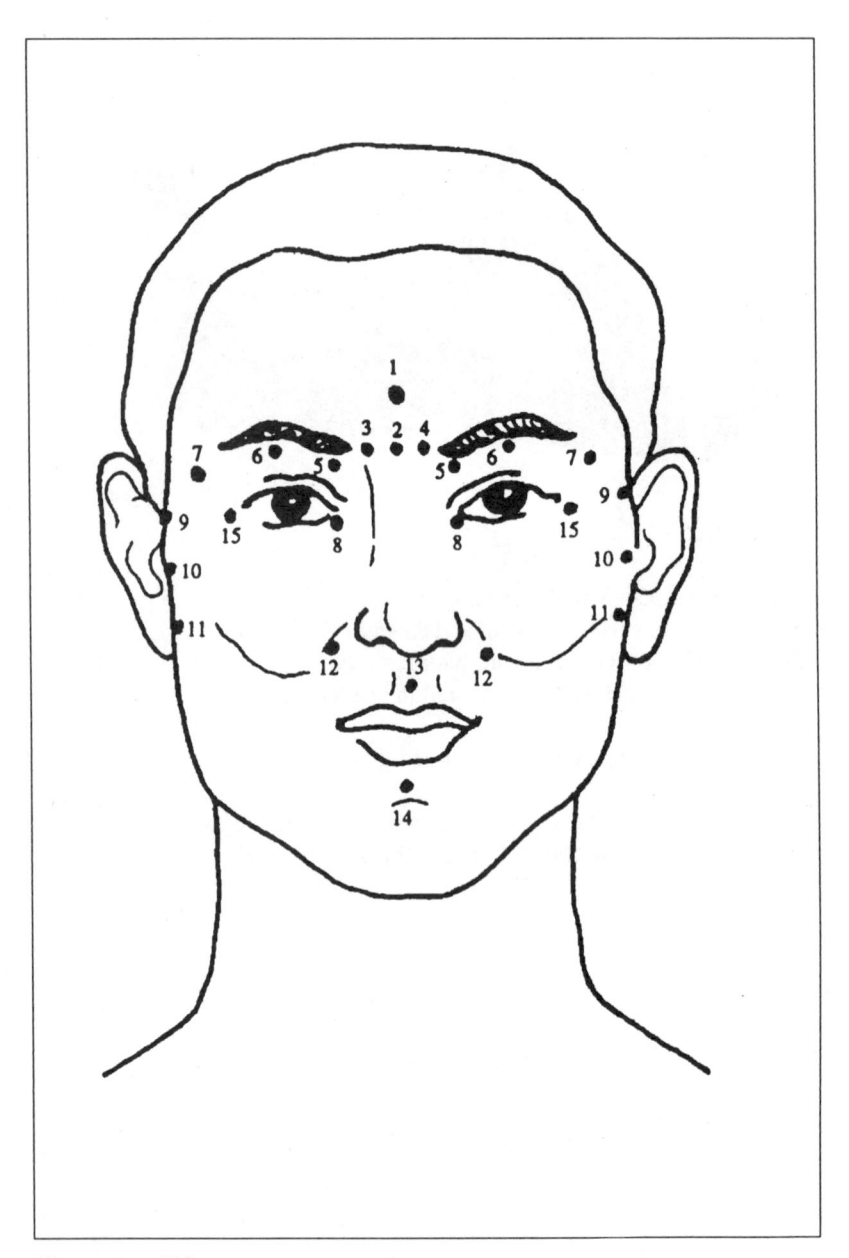

*Illustration 109*

*A Whole-body Massage*

## SOME IMPORTANT ACUPRESSURE POINTS ON THE FACE

Illustration 109 shows some important acupressure points which can be worked during face massage.

**Point 1:** The 'Third Eye'; in the Sanskrit terminology of Yoga it is called the Ajna Chakra. It is the sixth of the seven main energy centres in the body.

**Point 2:** Therapy point for headache, insomnia, problems of the lower sinuses, dizziness.

**Points 3:** Therapy points for headache and facial paralysis.

**Point 4:** Therapy point for headache and facial paralysis.

**Points 5:** Therapy points for headache.

**Points 6:** Therapy point for facial paralysis and hypothermia.

**Points 7:** The temples. One of the most important and effective therapy points for headache. Also for facial paralysis.

**Points 8:** The tear ducts. The best therapy for insomnia—and absolutely harmless, with no side-effects. Throw away your sleeping pills! Soft pressure on the tear ducts (sustained for up to one minute or more and repeated several times) is also excellent for relaxing the whole body. Only very gentle thumb pressure is necessary.

**Points 9, 10 and 11:** Small depressions next to the upper and the lower edge and the middle of the ear. Therapy points for deafness, ear pain, and toothache.

**Points 12:** Therapy points for problems of the lower sinuses and for facial paralysis.

**Point 13:** The 'unconsciousness point'. (An important point in Chinese acupuncture as well, where it is called 'Renzhong'). Therapy point for faint, shock, sunstroke, and respiratory failure.

**Point 14:** Therapy point for facial paralysis.

**Point 15:** Therapy point for migraine.

## HOW TO GIVE A FACE MASSAGE

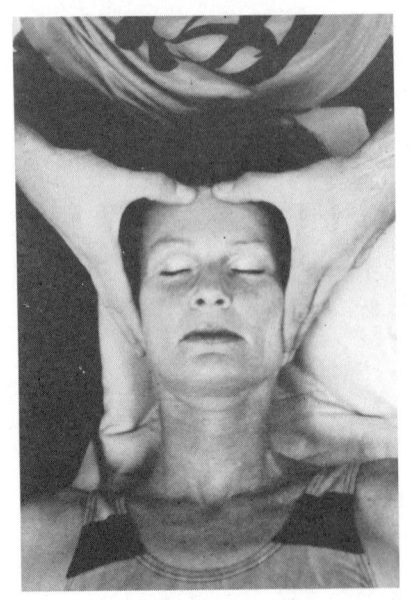

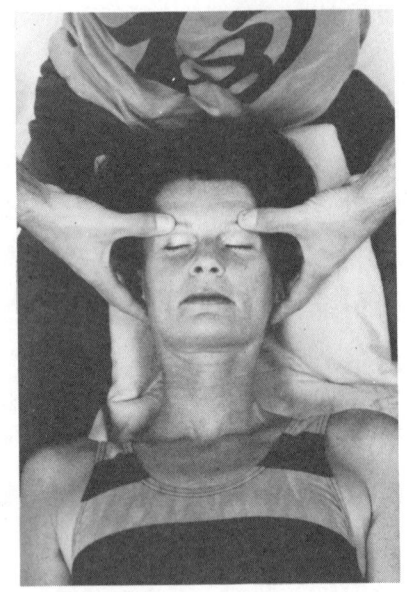

*Illustration 110*  *Illustration 111*

Sit behind the patient in a comfortable posture. Put a pillow on your lap and place the patient's head on the pillow.

For a good face massage you need a calm hand and a lot of sensitivity. The kind of face massage I give is gentle and calming. Some of my colleagues work quite rough and hard on the face. I see no point in that except in certain therapies where hard massage is necessary. Follow your intuition and your feelings.

The acupressure points introduced in Illustration 109 may be seen as a guideline. Start with caressing finger movements on the whole face. (Are your hands cold? Then rub them together to warm them up first.)

Illustration 110 and 111 give you an example of how to massage with your thumbs. Move your thumbs across the forehead and the eyebrows. Always work towards the temples.

**Caution:**  If you haven't checked before, ask whether the patient is wearing contact lenses. If yes, omit the following exercise.

*A Whole-body Massage*

Move with your thumbs around the eyes, covering Points 5, 6 and 15. Cover the tear ducts with light pressure (see Illustration 112).

Work along the upper and lower jaw with gentle pressure and with rubbing movements.

Play with the ears. (On the ears there are 115 acupressure points for the whole body.) Close the ears for 10-15 seconds, which is very relaxing. We can close our eyes when we are tired but when do we close our ears?

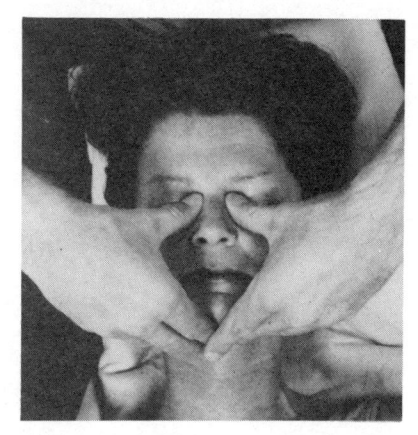

*Illustration 112*

Do caressing movements on and around the temples. Repeat parts of the face-massage as often as you like. And just use your imagination.

As the 'grand finale' I suggest that you hold the 'Third Eye' for at least a minute with very gentle pressure (Illustration 113).

You will be astonished how easy it is to create heaven on earth for your partner if you show a little bit of sensitivity.

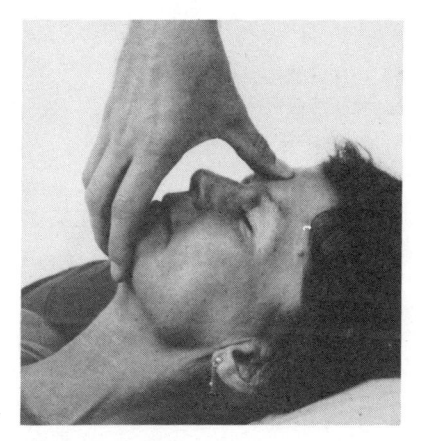

*Illustration 113*

# PART III

# APPENDICES

*Appendixes*

## 3.1 THE THEORY OF THE TEN *SEN*: THE ENERGY MAINLINES IN THE BODY

As mentioned in the introduction, the concept of the 10 *Sen* forms the theoretical foundation of Thai massage. It must be said, however, that there is more than one opinion about the actual running of the 10 *Sen* and various traditions place them differently. I've decided to give you a version that is used by many therapists and which I use myself.

Whoever is familiar with the Meridians in Chinese acupuncture or with the system of the Prana Nadis in Yoga will find lots of similarities. All the Chakras, the main energy centres in the Yoga tradition, are covered. I'm personally very much convinced that all these different traditions have the same origin and background and that the differences we find today are of minor importance. Anyway, whatever system of energy lines you use for your work, it is based on the experience of hundreds of years - and it does work.

While learning basic Thai massage, a detailed knowledge of the 10 *Sen* is not necessary. When doing the exercises in this book you are in fact frequently working on the lines without being aware of them and without me specifically mentioning them.

As we are not working on definable anatomical entities, the running of the lines described below can only be a guideline. Time and a lot of pratice is needed for the masseur to develop a feeling for the lines.

A workout specifically on the lines is essential for the therapist, but not for someone giving 'General Massage'. Nevertheless, a cursory overview of the therapeutic use of the lines is given below.

The main indications are given in bold print.

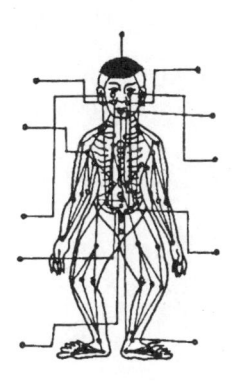

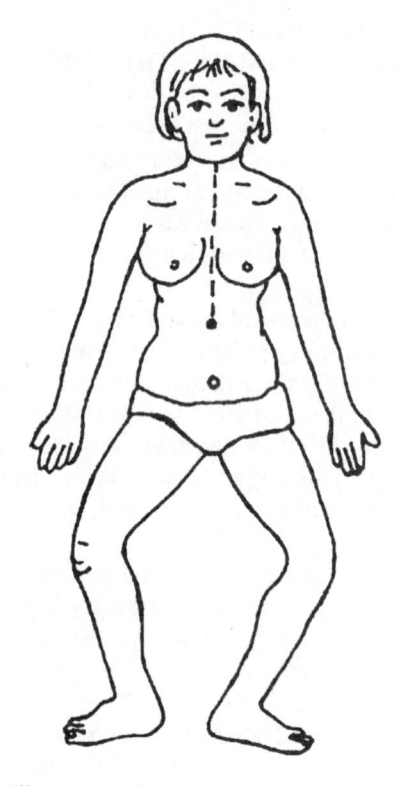

*Illustration 114*

## 1. SEN SUMANA

*Sen Sumana* starts at the tip of the tongue, travels down the throat and chest to the solar plexus. It's path is quite similar to Sushumna Nadi in the Yoga Tradition and also the Ren Mai Meridian in Chinese acupuncture.

**Therapy:Asthma, bronchitis, chest pain**, heart diseases, spasm of the diaphragm, nausea, cold, **cough**, throat problems, diseases of the digestive system, abdominal pain.

*Appendixes*

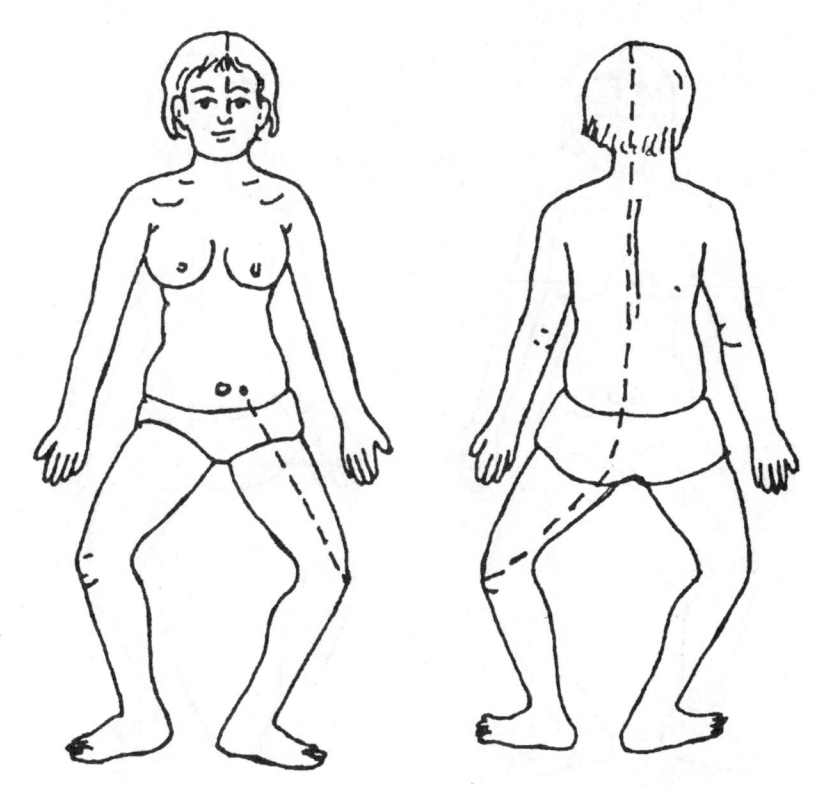

*Illustration 115*

## 2. SEN ITTHA

*Sen Ittha* starts at the left nostril, travels up to the head and down the neck. Becomes Line 1 on the back, crosses the buttocks and moves down the third outside line on the thigh. Changes then to the front of the body and becomes the first inside line on the thigh. Goes up to the abdomen and stops one thumb distance left from the navel. It is similar to Ida Nadi in Yoga and to the urinary bladder meridian in acupuncture.

**Therapy:** Headache, stiff neck, shoulder pain, common cold, cough, nasal obstruction, throat ache, eye pain, chill and fever, **abdominal pain, intestinal diseases, back pain, diseases of the urinary tract**, dizziness.

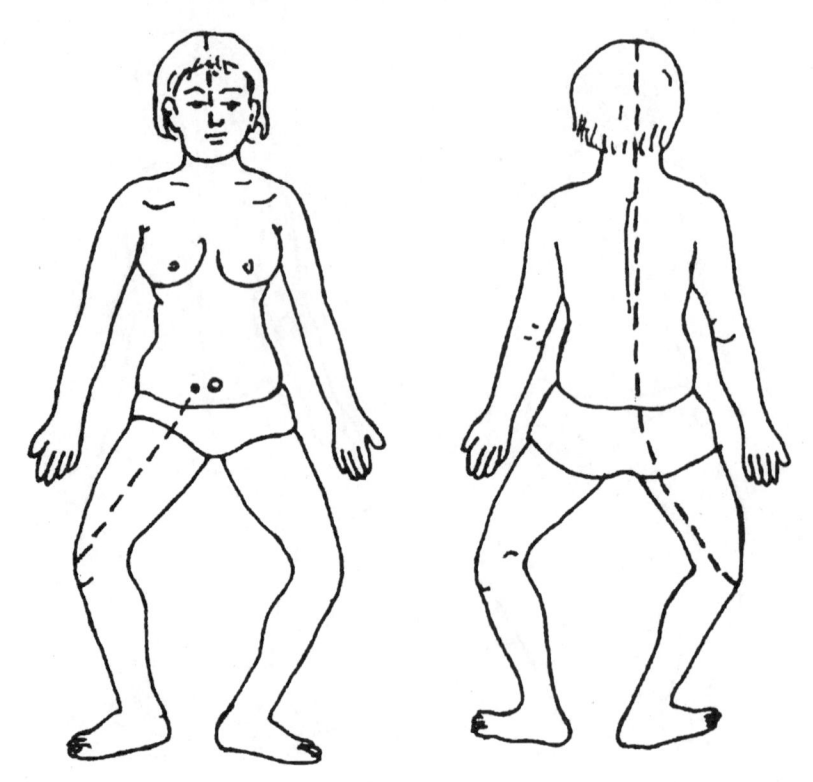

*Illustration 116*

### 3. SEN PINGKHALA

*Sen Pingkhala* takes the same course as *Sen Ittha*, yet on the right side of the body. Similarity to Pingala Nadi in Yoga.

**Therapy**: Same as *Sen Ittha*. Additional indications: **Diseases of the liver and the gall bladder.**

*Appendixes*

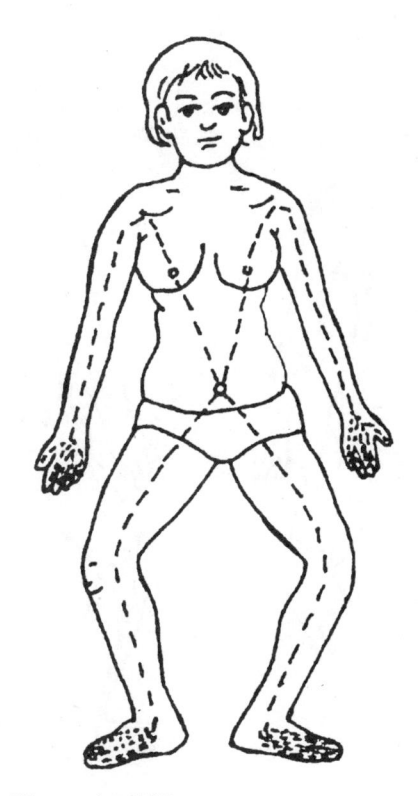

*Illustration 117*

## 4. SEN KALATHARI

*Sen Kalathari* starts at the navel and divides into branches, two on the right, two on the left. From the navel up through the chest and shoulder down the middle line of the arm to the hand. From there to the tips of all the fingers on both the left and right side of the body.

From the navel down the mid-line of the inside of the leg (the second inside line) to the foot. From there to all the toes on both the left and right side of the body.

**Therapy:** Diseases of the digestive system, indigestion, hernia, **paralysis of arms and legs**, knee pain, jaundice, whooping cough, arthritis of the fingers, chest pain, shock, **rheumatic heart disease and cardiac arrhythmia**, sinusitis, **pain in arms and legs, angina pectoris, epilepsy, schizophrenia, hysteria, various psychic diseases and mental disorders.**

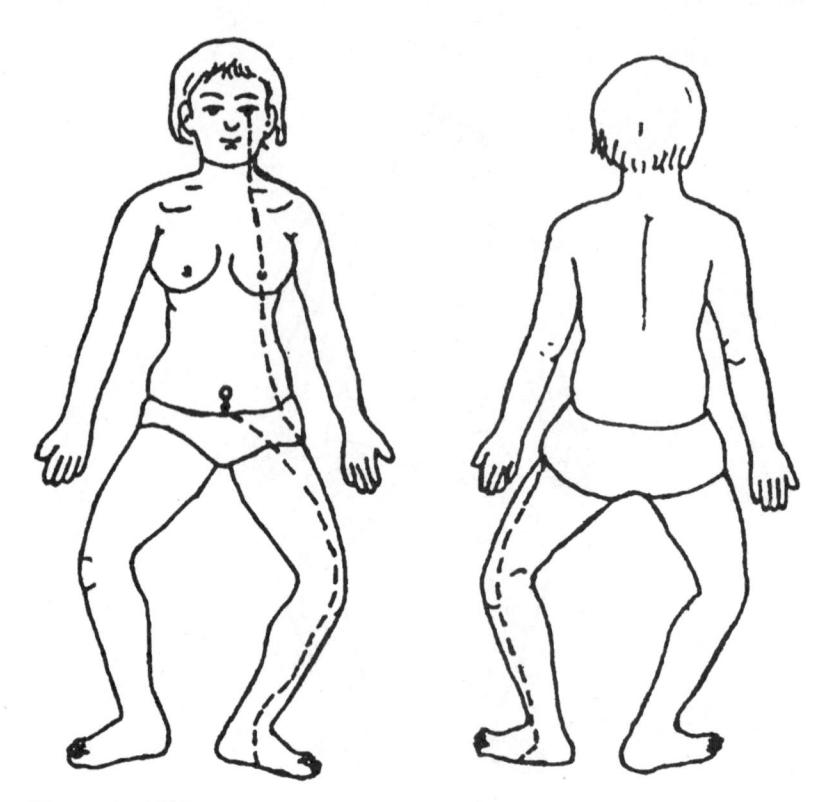

*Illustration 118*

## 5. SEN SAHATSARANGSI

*Sen Sahatsarangsi* starts in the left eye and travels down the head, throat, left side of the chest and abdomen, then changes to the outside of the leg coinciding with the first line on the outer leg. Changes again at the foot to the inside of the leg and forms the first inside line. This line continues across the groin and stops directly below the navel. It is quite similar to the stomach meridian in Chinese acupuncture.

**Therapy:** Facial paralysis, toothache, throat ache, redness and swelling of the eye, fever, chest pain, mania depressive psychosis, gastrointestinal diseases, diseases of the urogenital system, leg paralysis, **arthritis of the knee joint, numbness of lower extremity**, hernia, **knee pain**.

*Appendixes*

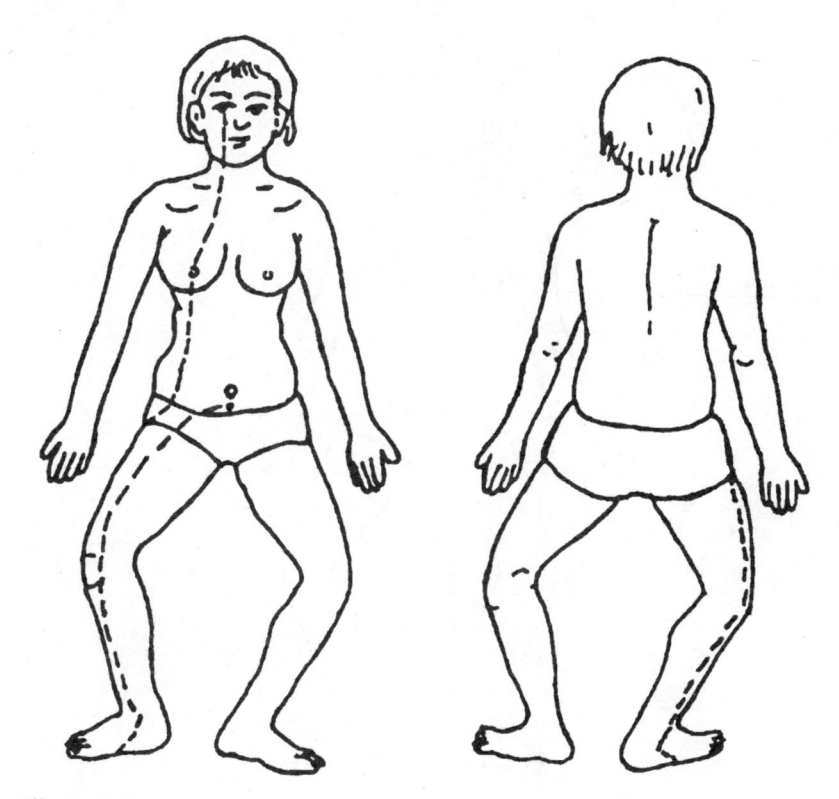

*Illustration 119*

## 6. SEN THAWARI

*Sen Thawari* takes the same course as *Sen Sahatsarangsi*, but on the right side of the body.

**Therapy**: Same as *Sen Sahatsarangsi*. Additional indications: jaundice and appendicitis.

*The Art of Traditional Thai Massage*

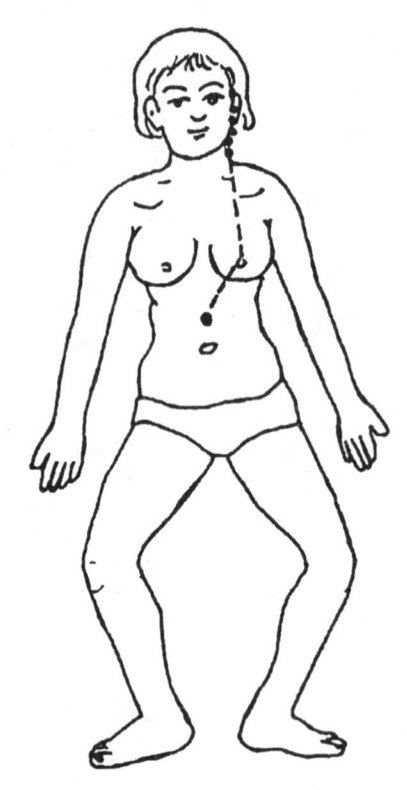

*Illustration 120*

## 7. SEN LAWUSANG

*Sen Lawusang* starts in the left ear, travels down the left side of the throat, then towards the nipple. Makes a slight turn thereafter towards the navel and ends at the solar plexus.

**Therapy: Deafness, ear diseases**, cough, facial paralysis, toothache, throat ache, chest pain, gastrointestinal diseases.

*Appendixes*

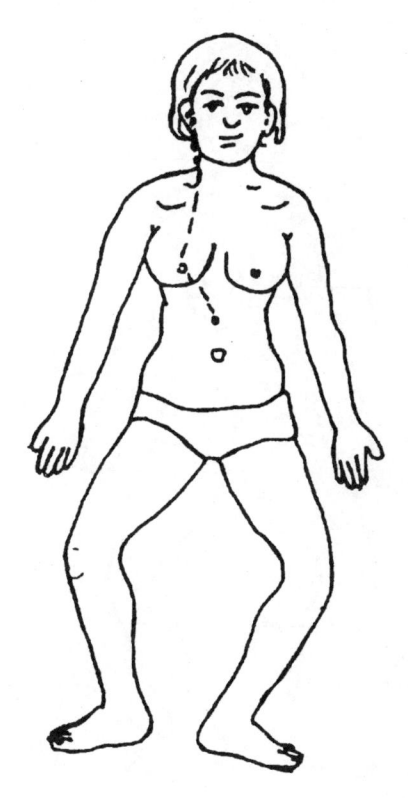

*Illustration 121*

**8. SEN ULANGKA** (Also called *Sen Rucham*)

*Sen Ulangka* takes the same course as *Sen Lawusang*, yet on the right-side of the body.

**Therapy**: Same as *Sen Lawusang*.

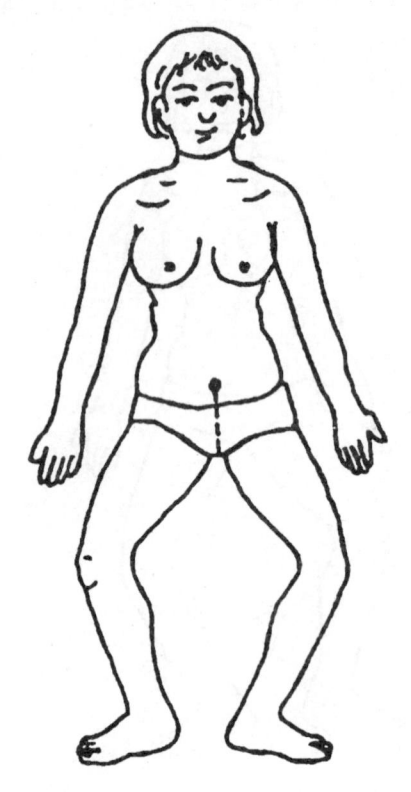

*Illustration 122*

### 9. SEN NANTHAKRAWAT

*Sen Nahthakrawat* comprises two lines:

> -Starts at the navel and runs as *Sen Sikhini* to the urethra or urinary passage.

> -Starts at the navel as well and runs as *Sen Sukhumang* to the anus or fecal passage.

**Therapy**: *Sen Nanthakrawat* is generally worked on by giving an abdominal massage. Indications are: hernia, **frequent urination, female infertility, impotence, precox ejaculation, irregular menstruation, uterine bleeding, retention of urine**, diarrhoea, abdominal pain.

*Appendixes*

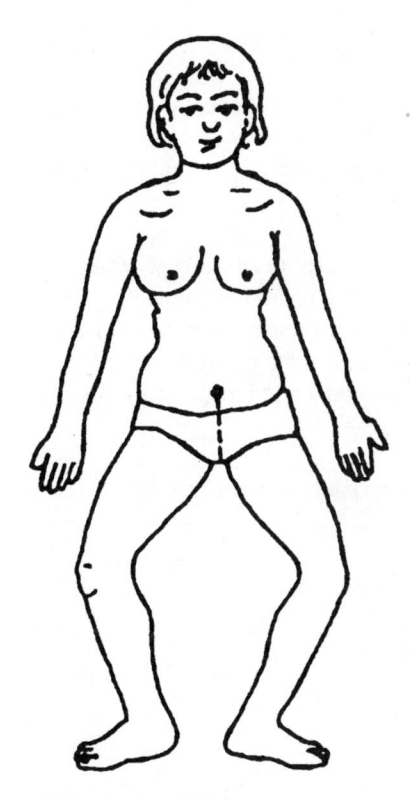

*Illustration 123*

## 10. SEN KHITCHANNA

*Sen Khitchanna* is broadly similar to *Sen Nanthakrawat*. It runs from the navel to the penis as *Sen Pitakun* (male) and from the navel to the vagina as *Sen Kitcha* (in women).

**Therapy:** Therapy on *Sen Khitchanna* is done with abdominal massage as well. Same indications as with *Sen Nanthakrawat*.

## 3.2 THERAPY

The techniques described so far in this book are sufficient for basic treatment for headache, knee pain and (lower) back pain. I won't introduce anything new in this chapter but rather show you how to combine the exercises already learnt to do simple therapies.

An important difference between therapy and general massage lies in the way you work. Start working the acupressure points with light pressure; increase the pressure each and every time you repeat. Generally you have to work harder than in a relaxing massage. Hold the points longer, up to 10 seconds or more. Take up to 10 minutes to work on the most important points relevant for the particular illness.

If the patient is in too much pain to receive pressure, first apply a hot wet towel on the area to be treated.

Repeat the therapy as often as necessary.

*Appendices*

## 3.2.1 HEADACHE

Headache may have many causes. The combination of exercises suggested here can alleviate a broad variety of possible causes.

Start with a foot massage, putting your main emphasis on the exercises shown in Illustration 15 and in Illustration 18, (points for sinusitis).

Work the arm line depicted in Illustration 63.

Do the set of exercises in 2.1.7 (Hands and fingers). Illustration 64 shows some important acupressure points, of which Point 1 as the main 'pain-killer' will especially be helpful. But it's best to give a full hand massage.

Quite often headache results from tension in the neck and in the shoulders. Do the set of exercises in 2.4.2 (arms, shoulders, and shoulder blades). Go through all the exercises of that chapter.

A multitude of acupressure points, as well as exercises, is mentioned in section 2.4.3. Head and neck, too.

Finish the headache therapy with Part 2.5 (The Face Massage). The headache points are described there in detail.

In most cases of headache you will either manage to cure your patient with this treatment or at least achieve noticeable relief.

*The Art of Traditional Thai Massage*

### 3.2.2 KNEE PAIN

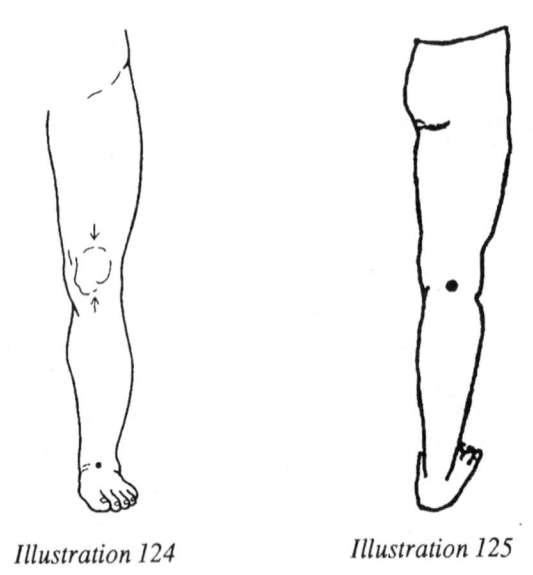

*Illustration 124*     *Illustration 125*

To alleviate knee pain, press and rub between the tendons on the dorsum of the feet, as explained in Illustration 16.

Press the point at the juncture of the foot and leg (shown and explained in Illustration 15 and depicted in Illustration 124). While pressing with one thumb, push the foot back towards the patient's body with your other hand, holding the toes and the ball of the foot. Repeat a couple of times.

Intensively work all the six lines on the legs with palming and thumbing. The most important of the six lines for relaxing the knee is the first outside line — work it several times.

With your thumb push the patella alternately up and down (Illustration 124).

In the position of lying on the side or lying prone bend the patient's lower leg and press with the thumb (or thumb on thumb) the point in the centre behind the patella (Illustration 125). Stretch the leg out and bend again.

This massage will help in cases of over-strain and overworking of the knee. In problems of the meniscus, cure is not possible with massage. Nonetheless, the techniques described here will give some relief from acute pain.

*Appendices*

## 3.23 LOWER BACK PAIN

For lower back pain start with working the lines on the legs, especially the third inside line on which there are several points for the back.

Continue with the stomach massage explained in Part 2.1.5. Pain in the lower back is often caused by tension in the abdominal region.

In the side position press the point behind the centre of the patella (Illustration 125).

Also helpful is to press the third outside line on the legs in the area of the painful spots around the pelvis and buttocks (see Illustration 68).

Then work both sets of back lines shown in Illustration 81. In the lower part of the back, below the ribs, do thumbing in the kidney area approximately one of your patient's thumb lengths away from Line 2.

## 3.2.4 THE USE OF OILS AND CREAMS IN THERAPY

For the therapies explained here the use of oils and creams is not absolutely necessary, but it's perfectly okay to use some oil after you have finished point pressure massage. If you use oil before, your thumbs and fingers will slip.

For relaxing muscular tension, my best experience has been with the Ayurvedic Mahanarayan Oil. It is easily available from Ayurvedic doctors in India, Nepal and Sri Lanka but might be difficult to obtain in the West. Possible alternatives might be coconut oil or sunflower oil. Tiger Balm or similar balms are good for headache and colds (massage the temples with it) but are also useful for tense and tired muscles.

Most 'Special Massage Oils' available in health shops and pharmacies are only plain oils which have been heavily perfumed; further, they are far too expensive.

*Appendices*

## 3.25 HERBAL TREATMENT

You may often find Thai massage being advertised as 'Herbal Massage' but in fact serious herbal treatment is rarely offered. In most places 'Herbal Massage' simply means that you have a herbal steambath before or after your massage. Some therapists, however, do use herbs to prepare hot, wet towels which are applied for treating muscular tension or warming up parts of the body that are too painful to work on directly. Many herbs can be used, including camomile, nettles, ginger, garlic, and many others. Sometimes masseurs use their own secret mixtures.

If you want to employ herbs for treating any particular problem, consult an Ayurvedic doctor and get his advice on what herbs you could use.

113

## 3.3 PLACES TO LEARN TRADITIONAL THAI MASSAGE

Thai massage is becoming increasingly popular. More and more places offer massage and introductory courses. The teachers and the quality of teaching may change, so I don't want to judge and recommend any particular place.

The six addresses mentioned below should be seen as a guideline only. Here are some suggestions of aspects to be considered while looking for a place to learn:

Does the place only offer lessons or do they give you the opportunity to practice what you have learned, preferably on different people? Practice is essential; lessons without hours and hours of guided practice are useless.

Be aware of money-making rackets, where 'Instant Thai massage' —lessons of a couple of hours only—are promised. To learn the basics of a full-body massage, a minimum of ten days is needed.

At present you pay about 2000 to 3000 Baht for an introductory course in Thailand.

If you don't speak Thai: Is teaching in English available? Or do they at least have a detailed instruction manual of their style in a language you can understand?

1. One established place where teaching in English has been available for several years now is the massage hospital of the 'Foundation of Shivago Komarpaj' in Chiang Mai, Thailand. This is the massage school where the author was trained. Nowadays they offer 12-day courses (taught in English) based on the Northern Style of Thai massage. Northern style in general is a bit more gentle than Southern style. Much emphasis is put on an intensive workout on the legs and the energy lines of the legs. (A common characteristic of Southern style is a frequent 'plucking' of the nerves, a technique hardly used in Northern style.) As this book is based on Northern style, the techniques and exercises are similar to those taught at the Massage Hospital, though there are differences in structure. After successful completion of the course, a certificate in basic Thai massage and a membership card of the Foundation are issued. Long term courses in massage therapy and in Ayurvedic medicine are offered as well, although in Thai language only.

   Address: "The Foundation of Shivago Komarpaj", Old Medical Hospital,
   near Chiang Mai Cultural Centre,
   Wualai Road, Chiang Mai.

*Appendixes*

2. Another traditional school of Thai massage and one of the most famous massage centers in the country is at Wat Pho in Bangkok, inside the temple compound. They teach the Southern style and offer 12-day courses. A manual is available in various Western languages, and a certificate in basic Thai massage is issued. The school at Wat Pho is a good place to enquire about massage therapy and traditional medicine as well.

    Address:   Thai Traditional Medical School, Wat Pho, Bangkok.

3. Courses based on this book are offered at the "rePlace" in Chiang Mai. 10-day classes can be booked.

    Address:   The rePlace
    Peng Sarnkam
    1, Chetuphon Rd.,
    Chiang Mai.
    Tel. 053/248-838

4. Another place which teaches Southern style Thai massage in Chiang Mai is in front of Wat Suan Dok. You can do a 10-day course there.

    Address:   Wat Suan Dok Traditional Massage
    in front of Wat Suan Dok, Suthep Road, Chiang Mai.

5. The author's main teacher, Chaiyuth Priyasith, is available for massage and teaching. As he does not conduct fixed corses, details have to be arranged individually. He practices Northern style, and though there are differences in techniques, this book could be used as a manual.

    Address:   Chaiyuth Priyasith
    52, Thapae Road, Lane 3, Chiang Mai.
    (Look out for sign "Massage").

6. Information on courses by the author is available from the following contact addresses:

    **In Thailand**: Asokananda
    G.P.O. Box 79,
    Chiang Mai 50000.

    While in Chiang Mai, enquiries may also be made at Sunshine Guesthouse, 24, Kaew Nawarat Soi 4.

**In Europe:** Asokananda
c/o Brust, Körnerstr. 5, W-7322 Donzdorf 3,
Germany

Information on Thai massage in Europe is also available at: "The International Society for Traditional Yoga- and Thai Massage", c/o Vera Lier, Angermunderstr. 45, W-4000 Düsseldorf 31, Tel. 0203/741382.

While in India information may be obtained from Bharat Mansata and Kusal Gupta at Classic Books, 10, Middleton St., Calcutta 700071 (Metro:Maidan).

*Appendixes*

## 3.4 GLOSSARY OF THAI, PALI AND SANSKRIT WORDS

| | | |
|---|---|---|
| Asana | S | A position in Yoga |
| Ayurveda | S | Traditional Indian medicine |
| Chakra | S | An energy centre in the body |
| Farang | T | A foreigner of European descent |
| Hatha Yoga | S | Physical Yoga |
| Metta | P, T | Loving kindness |
| Nadi | S | Channel, *see* Prana Nadi |
| Nuad | T | Massage, to massage |
| Prana | S | Life Force, Life Energy |
| Pranamaya Kosha | S | Energy-Body |
| Prana Nadi | S | Energy channel, energy line |
| Puja | P, S | Religious ceremony (worship) in Buddhism and Hinduism |
| Sangha | P, T | The order of Buddhist monks and nuns |
| Sen | T | Energy mainline in Thai massage |
| Siam | T | Thailand |
| Wat | T | Buddhist temple |
| Wai | T | To pay respect by holding one's hands in an attitude of prayer |
| Wai Khru | T | To pay respect to a teacher in a religious ceremony |

T=Thai          P=Pali          S=Sanskrit

## 3.5 BIBLIOGRAPHY

Association of the Traditional Medical School (in Thailand). *The Medical Texts which His Majesty King Rama III had engraved at Phra Chetuphon (Wat Pho) in B.E. 2375 (A.D. 1832).* Bangkok, 1977.

Boonthumee, Piched. *Basic Therapy Techniques.* 3/3 Moo Ban; Ban Chang Kum, Tambol Bahn Vehn, Amphur Hang Dong, Chiang Mai 50230, Thailand.

The Cooperative Group of Shandong Medical College and Shandong College of Traditional Chinese Medicine. *Anatomical Atlas of Chinese Acupuncture Points.* Jinan, China; Shandong Science and Technology Press, 1982.

Eyermann, Ken. *Massage.* London; 1987.

Fiske, Ham. *Just Another Myth.* Bangkok Post. 19.2.1989.

The Foundation of Shivago Komarpaj. *Manual: Thai Basic Massage.* Chiang Mai, Thailand, 1987.

Gitananda, Swami. *Yoga-Step by Step.* Pondicherry, India.

Goson, *Traditional Massage*, Welcome to Chiang Mai Magazine, January 15-February 14, 1987. (pp 32-33)

Heyden, Mary. *Manual Basic Thai Massage Course.* The Foundation of Shivago Komarpaj, Chiang Mai, Thailand. 1988.

Louberé, Simon de la. *The Kingdom of Siam.* London, 1693, Bangkok, 1968.

Mulholland, Jean. *Thai Traditional Medicine: A Preliminary Investigation.* Department of Indonesian Languages and Literatures, Australian National University. 1977.

Riley, James N. *Thai Manipulative Medicine as Represented in the Wat Pho Epigraphies.* East Lansing, Michigan; College of Osteopathic Medicine; Michigan State University. 1979.

Svoboda, Dr. Robert. *The Hidden Secret of Ayurveda.* Pune, India. 1980.

Thapar, Romila. *A History of India, Vol.1.* Penguin Books; Harmondsworth, England. 1966.

*Appendices*

## 3.6. THAI BIBLIOGRAPHY

กรุงไกร  เจนพาณิชย์, รศ. นพ.
*การนวด ถนอมรักษาสายตาด้วยตนเอง*
โครงการฟื้นฟูการนวดไทย, กรุงเทพฯ, พ.ศ. 2531, 8 หน้า

โครงการฟื้นฟูการนวดไทย
*คู่มือการนวดไทย ในการสาธารณะสุขมูลฐาน (พิมพ์ครั้งที่ 3)*
สำนักพิมพ์หมอชาวบ้าน, กรุงเทพฯ, พ.ศ. 2531, 140 หน้า ราคา 35 บาท
ISBN 974-87433-8-1

โครงการฟื้นฟูการนวดไทย,
กลุ่มศึกษาปัญหายา, มูลนิธิสาธารณะสุขกับการพัฒนา
*ร่างกายของเรา : พื้นฐานการนวดไทย*
สงวนลิขสิทธิ์โดยโครงการฟื้นฟูการนวดไทย, กรุงเทพฯ, พ.ศ. 2529
ISBN 974-87433-6-5 165 หน้า, ราคา......บาท

โครงการฟื้นฟูการนวดไทย
*สายสัมพันธ์ [ข่าวสาร]* ปีที่ 4 ฉบับที่ 4
เดือนเมษายน พ.ศ. 2532, 34 หน้า

จิตรา  สีสวรรณ  (แปล)
*จุด เล็ก เล็ก ของ นิด นิด พิชิตโรค*
*คู่มือการรักษาตนเองด้วยวิธีพื้นบ้านจีนโบราณ*
สำนักพิมพ์ นานมี, กรุงเทพฯ, พ.ศ. 2530, 95 หน้า, ราคา 30 บาท

ชุมพล  พูนยิ่ง
*กดกระตุ้นฝ่าเท้า รักษาโรคและเสริมสุขภาพตนเองแนวใหม่*
สำนักพิมพ์ ยินหยาง, กรุงเทพฯ, พ.ศ. 2531, 103 หน้า, ราคา 35 บาท

ประโยชน์  บุญสินสุข
*การนวดเพื่อความงามและสุขภาพ  ชุดแนะแนวสุขภาพประชาชน*
สำนักพิมพ์ เมดิคัล มีเดีย, กรุงเทพฯ, พ.ศ. 2530, 79 หน้า, ราคา 25 บาท
ISBN 974-87464-2-8

ประโยชน์  บุญสินสุข, นาฏวิมล  งามศิริจิตต์
*คู่มือการนวด ชุดแนะแนวสุขภาพประชาชน*
สำนักพิมพ์ เมดิคัล มีเดีย, กรุงเทพฯ, พ.ศ. 2531, 285 หน้า, ราคา 65 บาท
ISBN 974-73230-5-2

*ศิลปการนวดเพื่อสุขภาพ  ฉบับพิมพ์ ครั้งที่ 2*
สำนักพิมพ์ บำรุงสาสน, กรุงเทพฯ พ.ศ. 2531, 162 หน้า, ราคา 56 บาท
ISBN 974-245-6585

เสรี   อาจสาลี
*ตำราหมอนวด และยาแผนโบราณ, คู่มือสอบเป็นหมอแผนโบราณ*
สำนักพิมพ์ พิทยาคาร, กรุงเทพฯ, 208 หน้า, ราคา 50 บาท

สุวิทย์   วิบูลผลประเสริฐ, น.พ.
โกมาตร   จึงเสถียรทรัพย์, น.พ.
*การแพทย์แผนไทย, ภูมิปัญญาแห่งการพึ่งตนเอง*
โครงการฟื้นฟูการแพทย์แผนไทย, กระทรวงสาธารณสุข
กรุงเทพฯ พ.ศ. 2531, 281 หน้า, ราคา 45 บาท
ISBN 974-7951-92-4

มหาวิทยาลัยศิลปากร
คณะเภสัชศาสตร์, วิทยาเขตพระราชวังสนามจันทร์ จ.นครปฐม
เอกสารประกอบการอบรมเชิงปฏิบัติการ   เรื่อง *การรักษาสุขภาพโดยไม่ใช้ยา ฟื้นฟูศิลปการนวดไทย,*  17-18 เมษายน, 22 หน้า

*Appendices*

อนันตปีน, ผ.ล.
*ตำราหมอนวดแผนโบราณ รวบรวมจากของเก่าโบราณ*
ดวงดีการพิมพ์, กรุงเทพฯ, พ.ศ. 2495 [2526], 116 หน้า, ราคา 50 บาท

หลอ เจี้ยน หมิง [อดุลย์ รัตนมั่นเกษม-แปล]
*นวดกดคลึงคุณหนู การนวดเพื่อสุขภาพของเด็กเล็ก*
*การรักษาและป้องกันโรคในเด็กอ่อน ชุดดูแลสุขภาพ*
บริษัท นานมี จำกัด, กรุงเทพฯ, พ.ศ. 2531, 150 หน้า, ราคา 40 บาท

หลิว ซื่อ เซิน [วีระชัย มาศฉมาดล, แปล]
*ศิลปการนวดแบบพิศดาร ตำราการนวดประยุกต์แผนโบราณของจีน*
*ที่เรียนรู้ได้ด้วยตนเอง ชุด ดูแลสุขภาพ*
สำนักพิมพ์ ยินยาง, กรุงเทพฯ, พ.ศ. 2531, 183 หน้า, ราคา 65 บาท
ISBN 974-335-146-9

ปริญญ์ ปราชญานพร [แปล]
*แก้อาการปวดหัวด้วยตัวคุณเองให้หายได้ภายในพริบตา ตามวิธีที่เลื่องลือของ*
*แพทย์จีนแต่โบราณ ประยุกต์กับวิธีการแพทย์สมัยใหม่*
สำนักพิมพ์ สุขภาพใจ ชุดเสริมสุขภาพ, กรุงเทพฯ, พ.ศ. 2531, 118 หน้า, ราคา 30 บาท

สมบัติ ตาปัญญา [แปล]
*ด้วยมือแห่งรัก, ศิลปการนวดเด็กแบบอินเดีย [Loving hands]*
สำนักพิมพ์สายน้ำ, ชุดครอบครัวผาสุข, พ.ศ. 2527, 158 หน้า,
ราคา 70 บาท

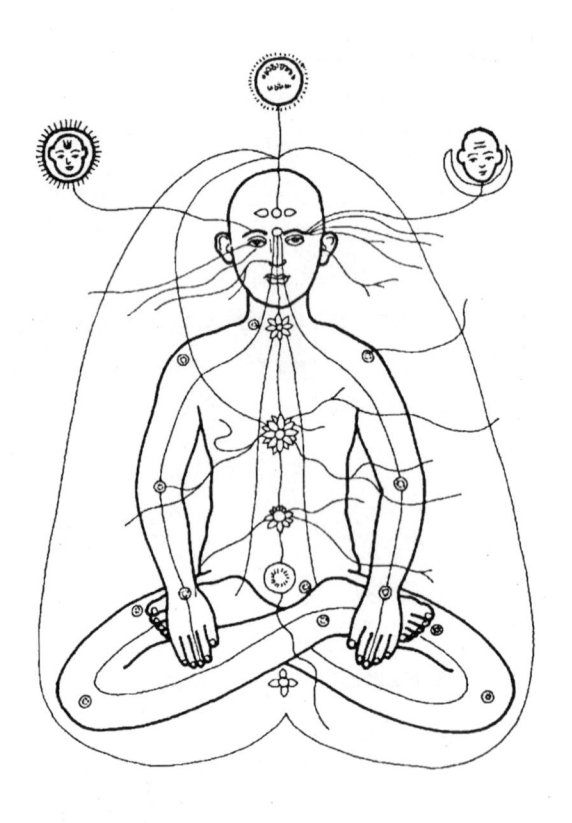

**New!**
**By the same author**
**"The Yoga of Mindfulness:**
**A Buddhist Path for Body and Mind"**